Bodystyling
beyond 40

Jutta Schuhn | Elmar Trunz-Carlisi

BARNES
& NOBLE
NEW YORK

© 2004 GRÄFE UND UNZER VERLAG GmbH, Munich

This 2006 edition published by Barnes & Noble, Inc., by arrangement with GRAFE UND UNZER VERLAG GmbH, Munich.

Photo production:
Marcel Weber

Additional photos:
Corbis: p. 2 (left), 6, 8, 13, 18, 25; Peter von Felbert: p. 26; Andreas Hörnisch: rear inside cover (Water); Manfred Jahreiß: p. 31, 43, 115; Jump: p. 11, 33; Manfred Kage: p. 17; Mauritius: front cover, p. 22, 46, 51; Nike: p. 55 (Shoes); Reiner Schmitz: p. 29, rear inside cover (yoghurt); Zefa: p. 45

Production:
bookwise Medienproduktion GmbH, Munich

Translation:
Sonja Marks

Important notice
The author and publisher have made every effort to ensure the information provided in this book conforms to national health and fitness standards and that the exercises are suitable for healthy individuals. It is not meant to replace the advice of a physician. Each reader is asked to make a personal decision as to which exercises are appropriate and how closely they want to follow the advice in this book. Neither the author nor publisher can assume responsibility for any injury, loss or harm resulting from the practices offered in this book.

ISBN (13) 978-0-7607-8496-9
ISBN (10)   0-7607-8496-5

1 3 5 7 9 10 8 6 4 2

Printed and bound in China

Foreword

We can sum up what's special about exercise after 40 in a few short words: it's worth keeping fit now more than ever!

It is precisely at this time of life that the body's capabilities decrease most significantly – looking at pure statistics. Often we experience something which does not necessarily need to happen: the years are reflected in our bodies. This is seen particularly clearly in the example of the musculature, which without targeted training will inevitably go slack. Because of this, posture, looks and not least your health all suffer. These processes of decline, however, are less a question of growing older and more the consequences of insufficient or incorrectly designed exercise. Since the body and, in particular, the musculature are just as "trainable" as before, you can maintain and even improve your fitness with no problem.

At forty you have settled into your lifestyle – and perhaps even feel more comfortable in your skin than you did at twenty. You can, however, still maintain your youthful energy for a long time to come!

For it to really work, your training concept must be designed to suit the particular needs and demands of women over 40. How to achieve the best results safely, effectively and enjoyably is what this book will tell you. At the heart of it all are the most effective body-toning exercises put together from the practical experience of over 20 years' teaching in the fitness field. You will be amazed at how quickly you will see success with this concept and how comparatively small the effort required is.

Jutta Schuhn
Elmar Trunz-Carlisi

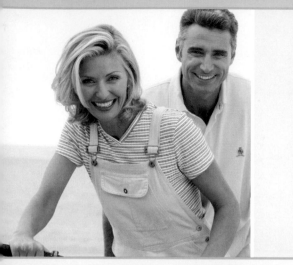
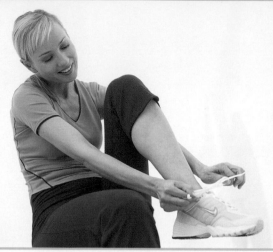

› INTRODUCTION

› PRACTICE

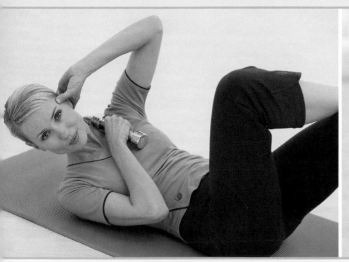
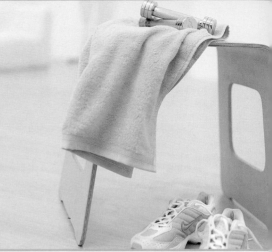

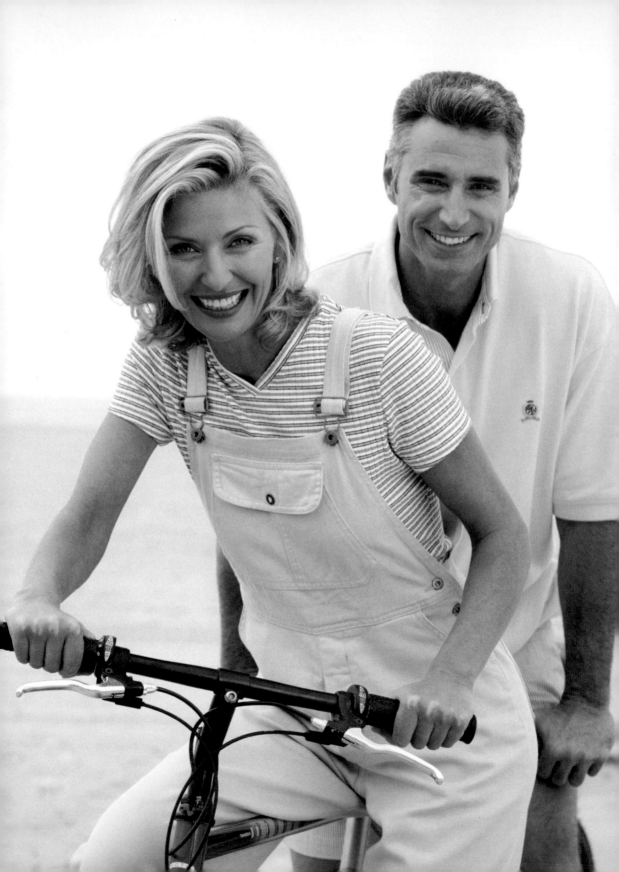

Start
today!

Women around the age of 40 find themselves statistically at about the middle point of their lives. So in front of you lie just as many years as you have already lived. Now is exactly the right time to set your course in terms of fitness. Those who live an active and healthier life can increase their stamina and keep going at a higher level for a longer period of time.

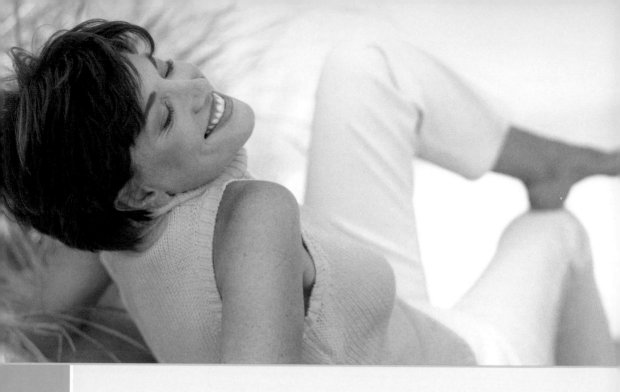

Your body is changing

Even if you keep yourself fit, changes will happen to you over the years – although fewer in your own body than in the overwhelming majority of other women your age. If, on the other hand, you do not exercise in a sufficiently targeted manner, increasingly you will find little deposits of fat building up where toned tissue and firm muscles previously defined your figure. Connective tissue starts to go slack. When buying clothes you can no longer get around the fact that you have to go up in sizes; many of your favorite clothes lead a half-life in the wardrobe because they are too tight or don't fit at all any more. Activities which you managed with ease in the past now make your out-of-shape muscles shake or your pulse race. Your back is also feeling the strains and pains more and more often. Added to all of this are the typical complaints of modern life, which are closely connected with an inactive and otherwise unhealthy lifestyle.

Setting your own biological age

It is a fact, verified by numerous scientific studies, that the process of decline described previously does not necessarily need to set in so early or take place so drastically. A decline in your health is not unavoidable. True, as a rule, most people actually experience a significant loss of capacity and chronic illnesses crop up more frequently. However, the majority of the statistical evidence puts this down to an inactive lifestyle, which is mainly characterised by a lack of exercise.

It is not your age as measured in years which is significant, but rather your biological age. You can judge this by how fit you are, how healthy you feel overall and not least by how young you feel. So the good thing about it is that you can set your own biological age to a large extent. You don't need pills, expensive treatments or any kind of miracle product. The fountain of youth is purely and simply targeted exercise together with a balanced, nutritious diet and a positive outlook on life.

Set your biological clock to "slow" – with an active life!

If you want to do something now for your figure and your health you should not only exercise regularly but also in a targeted manner. That is where this guide comes in. It contains, alongside important tips on nutrition and up-to-the minute fitness trends, highly effective Bodystyling exercises from which you can build a training program appropriate to your needs. You can tone your muscles to look their best and get rid of excess fat.

On the following pages you will find important information on which areas of your body now require particular attention. You will find information on how you can avoid all the fitness traps common in this phase of life. With an active lifestyle you can feel "just over forty" for many years to come.

The equipment

Your muscles, tendons, ligaments and joints are specialists in cooperation – if you do enough for them they will keep you young and healthy.

Just great: your muscles

Your muscles have to be stretched regularly so that they stay in shape. They lose basic tension and strength, become slack or over-strained if they don't get their exercise "high". Anyone who has had a cast for a longer period of time will know that a muscle forced to rest will lose almost all of its strength within just a few weeks.

But in everyday life, most of us fail to look after our muscles. Problems with the figure and posture are very common, particularly among "office types". They come about mainly because the muscles "atrophy" and the spine and joints can therefore no longer provide proper support. According to research, after the age of 30 muscle strength continually decreases. It has also been discovered that the amount we require our bodies to move around lessens to the same extent. The message is clear: loss of ability is caused to a great extent by an inactive lifestyle. If you regularly exercise your muscles you can mount a successful defense against the processes of physical decline – and put yourself significantly ahead of other women of your age. The amount of effort required is amazingly small, as the latest studies show: exercising two to three times a week for half an hour at a time is enough to produce clear results.

INFO

THE MUSCLES – ONE OF YOUR GREATEST ASSETS

Your musculature represents about 40 percent of your whole body mass and is thus your largest organ. You can put it to good use at any age. Your muscles represent the active exercise mechanism and, as opposed to the passive exercise mechanism (bones, ligaments and tendons), are well supplied with blood and therefore quite easy to train.

Teamwork: Ligaments, tendons and joints

The ways in which your muscles, ligaments, tendons and joints work are all closely connected with one another. Like fine ropes, tendons and ligaments in the form of taut bundles of fibres connect your muscles with your bones. They stabilize the joints and hold them in the optimal position. They also transfer the energy that arises from the movement of muscles to your bones, thus causing the joints to move. If ligaments and tendons are not sufficiently taxed, they increasingly lose their taughtness and elasticity. As they can now no longer sufficiently stabilize the joints, these

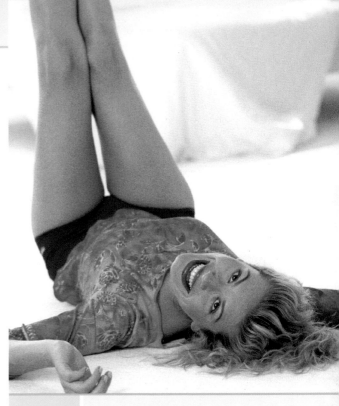

Your body is a finely tuned miracle of mobility.

become stressed and unstable – which is one of the factors that can lead to arthritis.

Apart from this, the cartilage acts as a protective cushion, absorbing the pressures caused by movement. The cartilage of the joints itself does not possess any blood vessels that supply it with nutrients. Therefore you have to get the cartilage pump going with sufficient exercise. This ensures that the important "synovial fluid" is always evenly distributed over the cartilage. With regular, targeted strengthening and stretching exercises you can successfully keep the signs of ageing in check.

Back and spine

Strong back muscles are good for your posture and your figure. They keep the body upright and thus show off the whole figure to its best advantage, particularly the upper body and chest. Other muscles that also have a part in this effect are firm abdominal muscles, which straighten the pelvis, and well-toned muscles in the region of the shoulder blades, which lift the breast bone and thus the whole upper body. You can encourage this "push-up effect" for better results with the exercises as shown on page 68.

Important buffer zone: Intervertebral discs

Just like your muscles, the discs of your spine also thrive on exercise. However they, unlike the muscles, are sparsely supplied with blood and get their nutrition from the metabolism of fluids. This pump effect, which occurs with gentle forms of exercise, is especially important for this metabolism. One example is power-walking, the gentler version of jogging: here the discs are gently massaged with every step. They absorb fluid – like a sponge – and thus remain lubricated and able to do their job. On the other hand, holding the same position for longer periods of time, e.g. when sitting, disrupts the discs' metabolic process and the tissues become brittle, losing some of their mass as a consequence. This makes the discs unable to properly fulfill their important role as shock absorbers.

Healthy discs – strong back. It's all a question of correct loading.

Strong together: Muscles and spine

If you include a weak or unevenly exercised musculature, then the vicious circle is complete; the muscles are no longer in a position to correctly support and stabilize the back. As a consequence, the natural curve of the spine changes, perhaps into a hunched back, which in turn encourages the sensitive discs to lock up. The resultant complaints can severely restrict your enjoyment of physical activity. Even if the body is generally able to keep these processes at bay for awhile, after 40 the back begins to rebel especially frequently and intensely. Not infrequently, it even results in a slipped disc, which is extremely painful. In the worst cases it can require a spinal operation. If you take care of your back with regular, well-balanced activity and targeted exercise of the muscles, you will most likely be able to protect yourself from these problems.

STRENGTHENING AND RELIEVING STRAINS ON THE BACK

TIP

The best strategy against a stiff back consists of a combination of regular light exercise, for example power-walking, and targeted muscle toning.

> Break up long periods of sitting with lots of short, active breaks. Change your sitting position frequently in order to spread the load on your back more evenly.

> Going for walks or power-walking promotes the supply of nutrients to the discs. Other forms of stamina-building exercise that are helpful here include jogging (only recommended for those of normal weight; pay attention to proper running technique!) or the use of a cross-trainer.

> Exercise the muscles of your waist regularly (page 86) and ensure that you balance the strength of back and abdomen.

> Maintain mobility with regular, gentle stretches. In the practice section of this guide you will find the appropriate instructions for doing this.

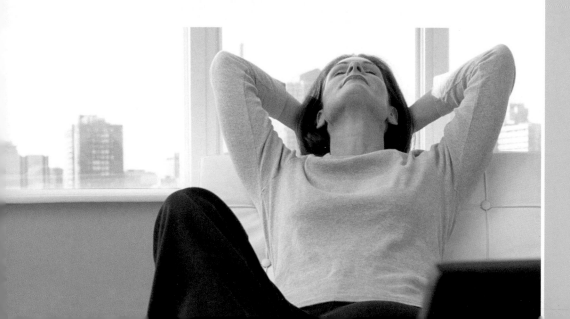

Connective tissue

When we consider connective tissue, one problem stands out in front of all the others and worries many women: orange-peel skin, or better known as cellulite. Cellulite is not an illness but basically a natural change in the female body. After a certain stage, however, it does present a real health risk because in the affected areas of the body the waste products of metabolic processes cannot be efficiently eliminated. A very high percentage of women are affected by cellulite in this country. How noticeable it is, however, depends on a number of various issues.

What causes cellulite?

There are three major factors mainly responsible for the appearance of cellulite: increasing fat deposits in the subcutaneous fatty tissue; slack connective tissue; and insufficient circulation to the affected body parts. The fat cells quickly increase in size and can no longer be sufficiently supported by the skin's connective tissue. Also, because the area is not adequately supplied with blood, waste products are no longer adequately carried away. After a while, the typical dimples and knots begin to appear underneath the skin's surface.

Only women are affected by cellulite because their connective tissue is more elastic and loose and is thus able to store more fat. The hormone estrogen is responsible for this and it also ensures that fat is deposited mainly in the problem areas of thighs and buttocks. However, this state of affairs does not reflect nature's blatant unfairness but has a purpose: The tissue would not be able to stretch sufficiently during pregnancy without the estrogen to make it soft.

It should not be ignored, however, that the tendency to produce cellulite is also a matter of genes. An inherited weakness in the structure of the connective tissue will make it more susceptible to cellulite.

One more thing: if you are a regular smoker, now is the best time to give it up. Stopping will not only be beneficial to your fitness, but will also create more favorable conditions for getting rid of cellulite: nicotine narrows the blood vessels, meaning that the tissue is less well supplied with nutrients and unable to properly eliminate waste products.

Red card for cellulite

If you know about cellulite then you already have the antidote in your hands. Even if the unwanted dimples don't fully disappear, you can still take concrete steps towards reducing them. Here are the key factors for success: Make sure that your fat cells do not get fed. Regular exercise helps your body to burn a lot of fat; a balanced diet will save on superfluous calories. This gives the fat cells no chance to grow – or to multiply. Fat cells, once formed, can be depleted by exercise and healthy eating but sadly they won't go away. The tricky thing about them is that the depleted fat cells are always signalling "hunger" to the body.

AM I AFFECTED?

Whether or not you have signs of cellulite or indeed how wide-spread it is can be determined with this simple test:

> **First signs of cellulite**
There are no superficial dimples. They only appear if you pinch your skin in the region of the thighs and buttocks between thumb and forefinger.

> **Advanced cellulite**
The typical orange-peel structure can be seen when lit from the side and when you tense the muscles in the affected areas.

> **Wide-spread cellulite**
Dimples and knots are clearly visible at all times on the skin's surface.

TEST

Toning the muscles in a targeted and controlled manner provides support for the tissues, encourages circulation and at the same time ensures that more muscles – and thus more "incinerators" – are available. In this way you use up more energy and store less fat.

In addition, anything that supports circulation is to be encouraged. Simple things such as a pulse-head shower or a skin-brushing massage are better than most expensive gadgets or cosmetics.

Hormonal changes

Around the age of 40, your hormone balance begins to shift, signalling the start of "the change". The change takes place over a long period of time and is individual and very different for every woman. First of all, the production of the hormone progesterone gradually decreases. Progesterone regularly prepares the lining of the womb to receive a fertilised egg. This reduced production causes the body to release more estrogen. This excess leads to more fatty deposits being able to accumulate in the subcutaneous tissues. As luck would have it, the appetite also increases after the age of about 45 when the production of estrogen finally slows down.

When estrogen levels fall, a further important change takes place: This hormone is what enabled the fertilisation of an egg in the monthly cycle. The monthly period now gradually appears less and less frequently. In their early mid-fifties women experience menopause, which marks the ultimate end to the cycle of menstruation.

Often connected with complaints

Because fewer sex hormones, in particular estrogen, are available to women going through the change, they experience a variety of complaints during this time. At the top of the list are disruptions in blood circulation to the skin (the well-known "hot flushes") and cardiovascular problems. Cholesterol levels rise and bone density decreases (see page 18). But it's not all about physical changes alone; the emotions often also take a hammering, and women may find themselves feeling unusually sensitive. Quite often women have to cope with nervousness and fear, sometimes even depression.

Exercise does you good all over

These natural biological processes can be positively influenced by an active lifestyle in many ways. It has been proven that physically active women show a lower rise in cholesterol and therefore have a lower risk of heart attack after menopause than women with a more sedentary lifestyle.

Targeted exercise also helps guard against osteoporosis (brittle bones, see page 18) or ease its effects. Especially appropriate here are the strengthening exercises around those areas particularly affected, such as the thighs, spine and upper arm. Positive effects can also be seen in the vasomotor symptoms (hot flushes) and in the reduction of fat deposits.

Launch with ease into a new phase of life

Exercise is especially good for the soul at this time of life, helping you continue to feel healthy, robust – and feminine. On the other hand, a positive attitude towards yourself can really help your body cope with these changes.

With exercise that is perfectly matched to your needs and a balanced diet, there is nothing preventing you from going through the change with élan and composure. Experience shows that women who make sure they do something positive for their bodies during this phase can even gain confidence, attractiveness and have a more positive aura. Many women even report increased spiritual clarity and a fresh outlook on life. See this new phase of your life as a chance and a challenge that you will rise to with verve, vim and vigor!

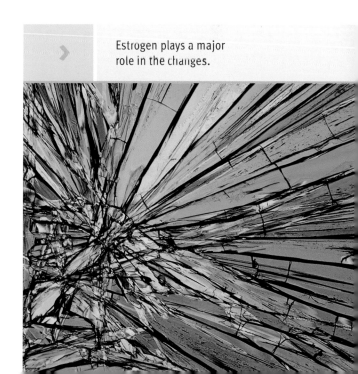

Estrogen plays a major role in the changes.

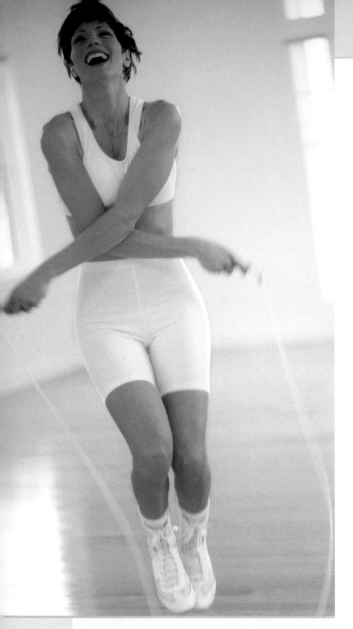

Don't be afraid to be "bouncy" – it's fun and strengthens your bones.

Bone density

Like all cells, our bones are constantly renewing themselves. The substance of our bones is continually being destroyed and replaced. These two processes are held in balance until around the age of 35. After this time, the process of destruction gradually takes over. It only becomes critical, however, when considerably more bone matter is destroyed than is normally the case. The bones become very brittle and become less stable. This condition is known as osteoporosis, when the bones become more porous, and brittle. With menopause comes a reduction in the production of hormones (see page 16). This means that the protective effect the sex hormones have on the bones and bone density is lost to a great extent in this phase of life. As soon as the hormone balance is restored after menopause, the process of destruction also returns to a normal degree.

Exercise is the most important protection factor

There are two particularly important factors for building up and maintaining bone density: a calcium-rich diet and, above all, lots of exercise. With regular, measured pushing and pulling exercises, such as those found in the practice section of this book, you can train your skeletal system and help maintain its stability for many years to come.

Particularly effective exercises to this end are those which require you to work intensively against gravity, such as step aerobics, for instance. Targeted muscle training also stimulates bone cells and ensures that you maintain a good figure – you should pay particular attention to the muscles responsible for posture. Strong muscles have the added advantage that they relieve pressure on the skeletal system and also protect it from injury.

It cannot be stressed enough just how important regular exercise is in preventing and treating osteoporosis. It is also understood nowadays that the first three decades of life are critical in determining how well bone density develops. The more active you have been and the greater the highest value of your bone mass ("Peak Bone Mass") over your lifetime, the higher the bone density "account balance" from which you can later make withdrawals. But don't think that it's just too late to do anything about the health of your bones; even if you only start your active strategy against bone depletion now, you can still considerably slow down the loss of bone mass.

Plenty of exercise and a calcium-rich menu – top strategies against osteoporosis

Exercise instead of medicine

Even in the medical treatment of osteoporosis, exercise and muscle toning are very important. There may be effective medications today which delay or even halt the loss of bone density, but hormone replacement therapy is not without its dangers. Side effects apparently include an increased risk of breast cancer according to the latest studies. Scientists therefore strongly recommend that such medication only be used in cases of extreme complaints during menopause – and then should only be taken for the shortest possible period of time. An active, natural prophylaxis against osteoporosis is even more important. It is never too early, nor too late to protect yourself with regular exercise.

How body tissue is put together

Over the years the amount of energy your body needs to perform its most important functions declines. So, if at 40 you are still eating as much as you did at 30, your body is programed to put on weight, as it no longer needs the same number of calories as before.

But even this process can also be influenced by a more active lifestyle. With every pound of muscle that you build up with exercise, the energy requirements of your body increase. It is the muscles that "burn" energy – even when you are at rest. This means you profit from your activity at any time of day – even when you are asleep.

A lack of activity makes itself especially apparent in your body composition – the relationship between fatty parts and fat-free parts of your body. From your 40th year at the latest, around one percent of your muscle mass is replaced by fatty tissue each year. You can only turn this very negative equation into a positive one with regular, targeted exercise.

When the scales lie

With scales alone you will only be able to poorly judge whether you have stored away too much fat. If, for example, you reckon your weight is "normal" or even "ideal" compared to one of the current charts (body-mass-index, Broca index), that is far from being a good reason to rest on your laurels. A body fat analysis, which is much more reliable, could show that your body fat quotient is too high.

In order to see your successes while losing weight, this method is very valuable. It allows you to continually check the amounts of fatty and lean tissue in your body. This way you will always know whether you have in fact lost fat or – as unfortunately is often the case for diets without an exercise component – if it is muscle mass that has been lost.

This is why many couch potatoes seem to be at their ideal weight despite having a body fat content above the recommended healthy levels. Similarly, fit and active people are sometimes classified as being slightly overweight. This is unfair, since muscle simply weighs more than fat.

Within the framework of a diet, this misnomer can lead to unnecessary disappointment. Those who lower their caloric intake and at the same time start exercising regularly will lose fat and possibly increase their muscle mass. If the scales show a more or less significant weight gain because of this, many give up in frustration even though they are actually on the right track.

Body fat analysis

There are various ways to measure your body fat. The most frequently used method is bioelectrical impedance analysis ("body fat scales"). The infra red method (in which the tissue is analysed with light) and the caliper method, in which the thickness of folds of skin are measured, have both proven useful. Charts of norms provide information about how the measured value should be judged; your age and gender are also naturally taken into account.
As a rule, the recommended body fat content for women is around 10 percent higher than that for men. There are different standards as women have greater stores of fat, particularly just below the skin. At the same time, in comparison to men, they have less muscle mass. Nature has, however, created a balance even here – women can tap into the greater fat reserves provided by their genes more easily than men can do. This assumes, of course, that they exercise regularly and concentrate on improving their strength and stamina through fitness (see page 41).

TIP

SIMPLE AND INFORMATIVE:
MEASURING YOUR BODY FAT CONTENT

If you don't want to buy your own "body fat scales", you can undergo a similarly useful analysis in any good fitness studio. Some health insurances also offer these kinds of tests. Along with your test results as a percentage, you will also find out how your results rank against the norms.

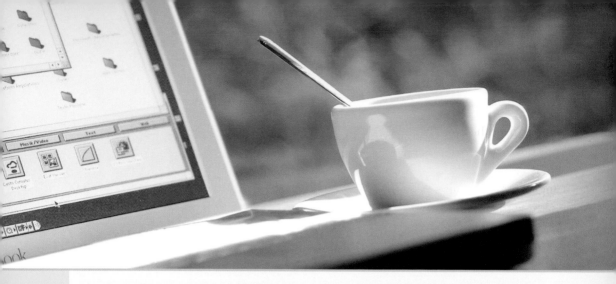

This cup of coffee with lots of sugar will wake you up quickly but is definitely not good for your metabolism!

Diabetes – the disease of affluence

The side effects of a sweet, comfortable life make themselves particularly clear if your metabolism gets out of whack. That's the case with type II diabetes, caused by obesity and is the fastest-growing illness of our time. In the USA the number of those affected has almost doubled over the past 30 years. Those most at risk are people over 40 who mostly work sitting down and eat foods high in sugar and fat. Other risk factors include nicotine and immoderate consumption of alcohol.

That's how easily diabetes can set in

When you eat, your pancreas produces insulin. This hormone distributes nutrients to all the cells of your body. Muscle, liver and fat cells have specialized receptors, onto which the insulin latches, allowing the cell to take up glucose (blood sugar), amino acids (protein) and fatty acids. If there is more sugar in the blood than the body's cells can use, the cells protect themselves from the excess of sugar in that the insulin receptors gradually give up their key function and, in the end, become insensitive to insulin. The sugar molecules now face locked doors and over a period of hours build up in the blood. The pancreas is thus forced to produce more insulin. Now, a portion of the sugar can be forced into the muscles, but the rest is carried away by fat cells and over the longer term is stored as fat. At the same time, the increased levels of insulin open up the gates of the fat cells, through which more cholesterol is taken up and "locked in" over several hours.

A high-fat diet can also cause insulin resistance. The insulin receptors become choked with fat from the inside of the cell outwards because the gates for the blood sugar are blocked up. Thus the vicious circle of lack of exercise, poor diet and insulin resistance is completed; type II diabetes is able to set in.

Tricky insulin

Your body is really quick to respond when it has too much sugar to deal with – for example, if you frequently eat sweet snacks. High levels of insulin are immediately ready to make use of the excess energy and store it as fat. The same is also true, by the way, for quick-burning carbohydrates such as those found in products made from white flour or in fruit juices with added sugar. Unfortunately, insulin also ensures that the fat cells remain "shut down" over a period of several hours so that the fat cannot be directly burnt off again. This is why insulin has recently been described as the fat-maker hormone.

HOW TO ESCAPE THE INSULIN TRAP

> Make sure that you experience as few "sugar highs" as possible with a balanced and regular diet.
> You will use more energy and keep your insulin receptors working normally with regular exercise. While on this topic, every-day exercise is also well worth the effort. Every extra step counts.
> When exercising, the most suitable activities are those which are not too strenuous that are performed over a longer period of time. These kinds of exercises are particularly good for your fat metabolism and create better conditions for reducing fat deposits.
> For those who are out of shape, power-walking is a great prescription.

IMPORTANT

Veins need exercise too

The veins leading to the heart could, during your lifetime, become varicose. This is especially true for the surface veins of the legs, which become enlarged and elongated, bulging out in wiggly lines. Not only does this look unattractive, it can also be an indication for health problems and other dangers. Women are particularly affected, since female sex hormones ensure that they have thinner connective tissue than men. This becomes particularly clear in pregnancy, during which around a third of women develop varicose veins. In the majority of cases these disappear after delivery. As you get older you will become more susceptible to varicose veins since your veins lose elasticity. Genes can also play a major role.

A healthy lifestyle can be especially successful in helping prevent problems with the veins. Among other things, nutrition and avoiding smoking can both play an important role. You should also make sure that your clothing is not too tight, as this can slow down blood flow. But there is one deciding factor that is more important than all the others – how frequently you use your muscles.

Exercising your blood vessels will keep your veins fit

Veins are a sophisticated network of vessels which are "powered" with help from the arteries on the one hand and the leg muscles on the other. "Fresh" blood, enriched with oxygen and nutrients, flows along the arteries in pulsing waves through the body. The veins, in contrast, have the job of transporting the "used" blood, laden with carbon dioxide and waste products, back to the heart. The pulsing waves in the arteries cause the veins to be regularly pressed together as well – a mechanism that is also known as the arterial pump.

Alongside this, the activity of the legs – particularly the calf muscles – is responsible for making sure that the blood in the veins can be transported upwards. There are valves in the veins that ensure the blood cannot flow backwards. If this important venal pump is not sufficiently activated, blood collects in the legs. Over a period of time the vessels become overstretched and bulge outward, which in turn prevents the valves in the veins from closing properly. The blood in the blood vessels now really gets backed up. The importance of regular exercise for the health of your veins becomes very clear if we take a look at early studies of people who had a more rustic lifestyle. They almost never suffered from varicose veins. This is mainly a result of their active lifestyle in addition to a diet consisting of naturally available foods.

Fitness for your legs

So, activate your leg muscles to spare yourself vein trouble. Gentle sports such as power-walking, jogging, swimming, cycling, step-aerobics or targeted fitness training for the legs are best suited to this purpose. In your everyday life there are important "rules" for the health of your veins: make sure you change the pressures on your body frequently. Try to avoid being in the same position for long periods of time or repetitive movements. Good ways to balance things out, for example, are short "activity" breaks – preferably with your legs raised. Especially try to avoid sitting down for long periods of time because the veins are pinched at the knees, which causes additional restrictions to blood flow.

 Keep it flowing ... treat your veins to a frequent "breather".

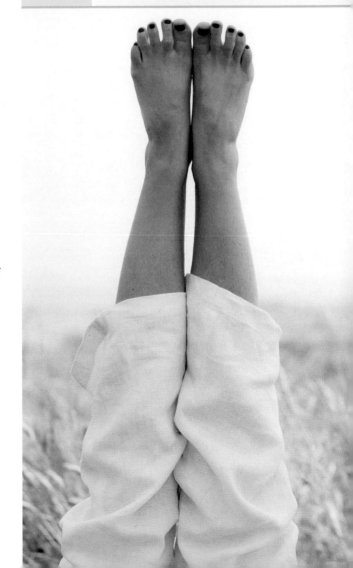

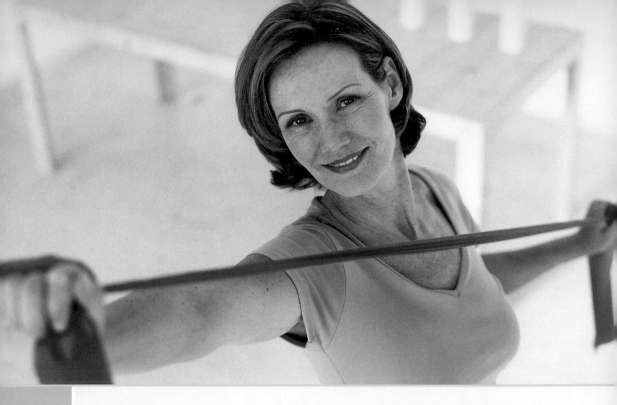

Collect body-forming bonus points

OK, so exercise, fitness and a good figure are easier for most people at 20 or 30 than for those at 40 or 50. The body is at its peak in its younger years; the payback for the little sins of nutrition or a lack of exercise are generally less noticeable at first and often only become obvious in later years.

But perhaps you yourself have already begun to notice that there are more and more women over 40 who are fitter and more able than many of the "young things". Age seems to pass them by almost without a trace. Their bodies and their whole presence radiate attractiveness and fitness, while younger women are already showing premature signs of aging. The age factor is therefore a really weak argument when talking about fitness, appearance and a good figure. The secret is exercise!

Activity keeps your body in shape – in the truest meaning of the word. With targeted exercises and the right training concept you can shape your body and also increase and protect your health. Both are especially important after reaching the mid-point of your life, since now is when you really have to set the course for your future. An active lifestyle ensures that you stay biologically young. A passive and lethargic daily life, on the other hand, will speed up the processes of decline that we all fear.

Do you know about vitamin M?

The advantages of well-toned muscles cannot be praised highly enough. Once again, here are the most important positive points about muscle-toning.

Toned muscles firm up the tissues

This is especially clear in the example of the abdominal muscles. Everyday activities are nowhere near enough to keep these muscles, so important for posture and figure, in top form. Without targeted training, over time the abdomen loses its basic tension. The stomach expands outward, fat deposits already present lose even more of their taughtness and become even more obvious. Specialized exercise will raise the base muscle tone and also firm up the surrounding tissue. By the way, the targeted, controlled exercises that you will find in the practice section of this book are particularly good for firming the connective tissue. These are exactly what you need to properly deal with cellulite (page 14).

Push-ups show off your figure to its best advantage

With specific exercises you can also drastically improve your posture. Most people who sit down a lot, for example, have a curved posture – the shoulders are pushed forwards, the back is rounded, especially around the upper spine. The whole figure suffers as a result of this, with the bust being drawn down by gravity instead of being lifted up by the ribcage, as just one example. You can support this straightening effect of the ribcage substantially by building up the muscles in the shoulder and upper back area, particularly the rotators and muscles of the shoulder blades. Because it is these muscles that ensure the ribcage lifts, the shoulders are also drawn backwards and thus your whole posture becomes more erect.

Muscles make you slim – around the clock

Muscles are the incinerators of your body. The more of them you have, the more calories you use – when working as well as at rest. Every extra pound of muscle means a significantly higher energy usage, which makes controlling your weight and your figure much easier in the long run. This does not mean that you have to look muscle-bound like a professional athlete. You will simply have more muscle tissue to call on, while others – often even if they have the same body weight – will have more fat to lug around.

Protection for the back and joints

Weak or unevenly developed muscles are not up to the important task of stabilizing and relieving the back and joints. It is estimated that around 80 % of all back complaints begin with muscular weakness or imbalance. Looked at another way, symmetrically developed muscles provide optimal active protection against premature wear and tear on the joints.

Your extra portion of health

We have already seen the benefits that regular exercise offers. Here are a few of the highlights again.

Avoiding the insulin trap

If you exercise regularly and also have your diet under control you will – unlike millions of other people of your generation – be protected from type II diabetes, the sugar-induced disease of the obese. With an active, healthy lifestyle you will create the best conditions for keeping your metabolism in rhythm and functioning at its best; you won't get caught in the infamous insulin trap (see page 22).

Controlling blood pressure and cholesterol the natural way

Of course you already know that elevated blood pressure and a high cholesterol count are risk factors for cardiovascular diseases. This makes it all the more important to be aware of effective protective measures. Regular exercise – particularly moderate stamina training – can lower your blood pressure or help keep it under control. Cholesterol can also be positively influenced in most cases, with regular exercise, avoiding smoking and using vegetable oils instead of animal fats. In this way the ratio of dangerous LDL and protective HDL cholesterol can be maintained or even restored. The more these two protein/fat combinations are in balance, the lower the risk to the cardiovascular system.

Burning fat – particularly effective for women

Compared to men, you possess around 30 % more body fat. The female metabolism though, to balance things out, is much better designed to burn fat. This means that you can tap into your fat reserves more easily and that you should be able to do this in a more targeted manner. In this respect, the best suited forms of exercise are light to moderately intensive ones, such as power walking, jogging or other stamina sports. The decisive factor is that you do not exercise too intensively, don't end up gasping for breath while training or allow your pulse to race (see page 43). Physically demanding activities in your everyday life – gardening is a good one – are also worthwhile over the long-term.

Effective protection against osteoporosis

Your bones need regular, measured push and pull loading (see page 18). Therefore exercises and movements which require you to use your body weight in a controlled manner against the force of gravity are particularly well-suited for this. Well-trained muscles are significant here too, because they surround bones and joints like a sturdy, protective sleeve. They effectively protect your skeleton from strains and breaks. The earlier you begin exercising, the greater the protective effect in later years.

That special lust for life

The spirit also benefits from regular workouts in a special way. Just like your muscles, confidence and a positive attitude toward life are also something you can both train and improve!

Turbo-boost your self-confidence

There is rarely a better opportunity to focus intensely on your own body than when you are exercising. Listen to your body and take note of its reactions and signals. With time you will be able to see more and more results. Having control over your own body, and over your posture and figure, will give you self-confidence in every aspect of your life.

Add years to your life ... and life to your years!

Everyone wants to live longer – but no one wants to grow old. But why not? With a healthy, active routine your quality of life can be maintained well into old age. Here and now the conditions for a long life have never been so good. But it can only be exploited and enjoyed by those who are still fit and independent in their old age. Targeted exercise is without doubt the best and most favorable way to accomplish this!

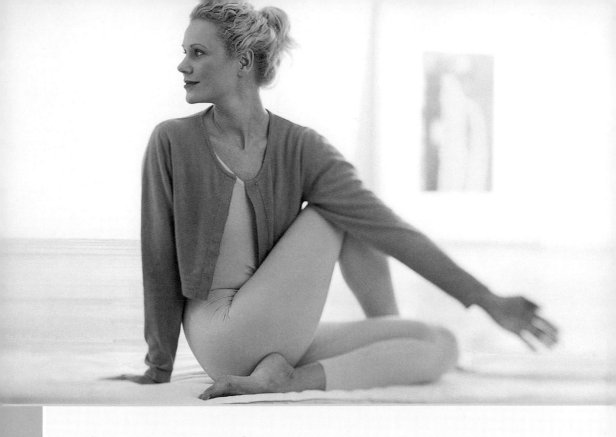

Classes and fitness trends

In modern sports and fitness clubs you will find a wide and varied range of classes to supplement your workout with targeted muscle-toning exercises. They can help you to build up your strength, stamina, mobility and coordination (from page 40) in a fun way. The nice thing about it is that you are always in the company of like-minded people. Have a look at the numerous classes on offer for whatever tickles your fancy at that moment and seems appropriate to your current level of fitness.

On page 35 you will find an overview of current sporting trends. You can see from the table at a glance what each of the fitness trends and classes listed on the following pages can offer you in terms of strength, stamina, mobility and coordination.

The gentle wave

The following selection of classes is particularly appropriate for beginners and fans of gentle, harmonious exercise. That doesn't mean that you can't push yourself while doing them …

Aerobics

Since Jane Fonda popularized aerobics in the 80s, aerobic (fat-burning) exercise has been a solid part of our fitness world. Over the years, though, the content has changed, and very much for the better. While earlier little attention was paid to the load on the joints, today the exercises are much more joint-friendly and are performed in a more measured manner. However, the less experienced and especially those who are overweight should only choose "low-impact classes", in which gentle exercises protect the joints from the hard knocks they would receive in the higher impact-versions. With correct, gentle exercise techniques aerobics can even help with back problems, as has been shown by sports science studies. Step-aerobics has the specific advantage that you are exercising particularly intensively against the force of gravity, which is especially effective at preventing osteoporosis.

Yoga

Exercise with an element of meditation is booming. Classical Indian yoga in particular is experiencing a renaissance in the fitness world. Yoga classes are not only good for physical fitness; the harmonious unity of body, mind and spirit – all-around exercise – promotes mobility and the capacity for concentration and relaxation, among other things.
You should learn the special breathing and exercise techniques from an experienced, competent yoga instructor. Beware of the popular "do-it-your-self" videos – the exercises and poses are often demonstrated too quickly and to imprecisely, which can lead to back strain and joint strain as well as to painful muscle injuries when you try to copy them. If you want to learn real yoga, you will need some measure of patience and you will also have to work intensively with your own body.

Power-Yoga

A very popular variation on classic yoga at the moment is power-yoga. As the name suggests, elements of fitness training are combined with meditative content in this new training concept. An interesting mix, especially for those for whom conventional fitness training is too functional and classic yoga too calm. The gentle but nevertheless quite taxing workout offers a synthesis of strength and mobility training. The class focuses on training concentration, physical control, breathing technique and relaxation.

Nordic walking

This form of sports walking with special poles is the natural progression from power-walking. While with that energetic form of walking the joints are under considerably less strain than with jogging, the addition of poles offers optimum joint relief. Nordic walking is also so popular – and with good reason – because it uses almost all the major muscle groups. This can burn especially high amounts of calories. Nordic walking is an all-around healthy and effective way to enjoy keeping fit.

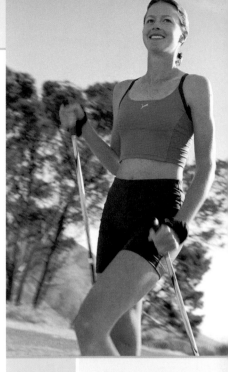

Nordic walking: ideal fitness training for all. Fun-factor included!

Pure energy

The fitness classes described below are also suited for beginners if they are performed at an appropriate level. But here we get a little more to the heart of the matter.

Pilates

This currently very popular concept was developed at the beginning of the 20th century by J.H. Pilates. The muscle-training exercises were originally meant for professional dancers – so for in-shape people who already had a particularly good understanding of their bodies. Even though the concept has been adapted for the leisure sports market in the meantime, some exercises should still be performed with care. With good Pilates instruction you can intensively and comprehensively strengthen your muscles. At the same time you can train both your concentration and posture.

Weight training

When you think of weight training you perhaps first think of bodybuilding. But if you find a good instructor and don't choose weights that are too heavy it can offer an effective fitness workout for you too. The accent is on strength and stamina, which brings many benefits for toned muscles as well as making for a good figure. The class concept is also suitable as preparation for those who later want to move on to professional fitness equipment.

Spinning/Indoor cycling

Group training on spinning bikes has become a discipline unto itself in fitness circles. You pedal virtual routes up and down hills to up-beat music. Even dedicated cyclists enjoy spinning as the movement involved is much closer to real cycling than previous static cycle-trainers. Good instructors make sure that your pulse doesn't race too much so that you don't overtax yourself, yet still effectively and specifically activate your metabolism of fat.

Tae Bo/Fighting Fit

In Tae Bo, typical moves from the field of Asian martial arts are put together with sequences from aerobics. As opposed to genuine martial arts, there is no partner work here and accordingly no body contact. If you want to improve your strength, stamina, mobility and coordination, enjoy overtones of Asian martial arts and like fast-paced sequences, you will really be able to get powered up for this style of training.

OVERVIEW: CLASSES AND TRENDS

Class	Characteristics/Suitability	Fitness benefits*			
	Points to note	Strength/Stamina	Mobility	Stamina	Coordination
Bodystyling	Suitable for all, generally even for those with joint problems.	●●●●◖	●●◖	●	●●
Aerobics, Step aerobics, Cardio-dance, Dance-aerobics, etc.	Choose suitable level. With weight and joint problems, low-impact classes only (see page 32).	●●●● (especially legs)	●●◖	●●●●●	●●●●◖
Yoga Power-yoga	The exercises should be taught slowly and systematically. Be careful with back problems.	●●	●●●●●	●	●●◖
Nordic walking	Optimal healthy exercise for all. Look for good equipment.	●●	●	●●●●●	●●
Pilates	Only with qualified instruction. Be careful with back problems!	●●●	●●●●◖	●	●●●
Pump Lift Weights	Exercise experience and good level of fitness advantageous. Build up weights slowly by building muscles!	●●●●●	●●	●	●●
Spinning Indoor cycling	Choose appropriate level. Start slowly. Keep pulse under control!	●●●◖ (legs)	●◖	●●●●●	●●
Tae Bo Fighting Fit	Recommended for all. Not too intense at the start!	●●●	●●●◖	●●●●◖	●●●●●

* The more dots, the more benefit you will feel from that form of exercise in the respective area.

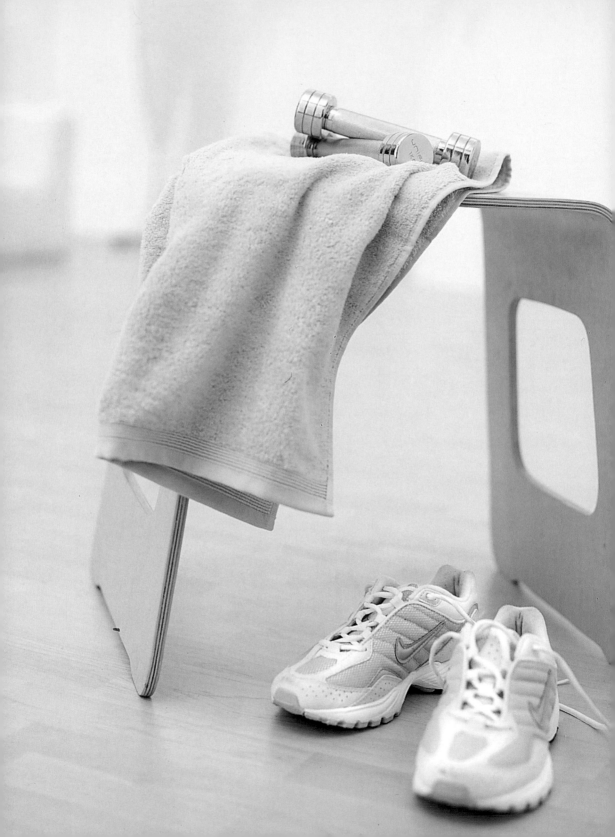

Your
workout basics

Before you get going, you should get to know a few important basic facts about exercise. Putting together the optimal workout for yourself is vital to ensure long-term success. Diet and – very important – your body's fluid levels are also involved in keeping you healthy, fit and attractive. In this chapter you will find lots of valuable tips for your training program.

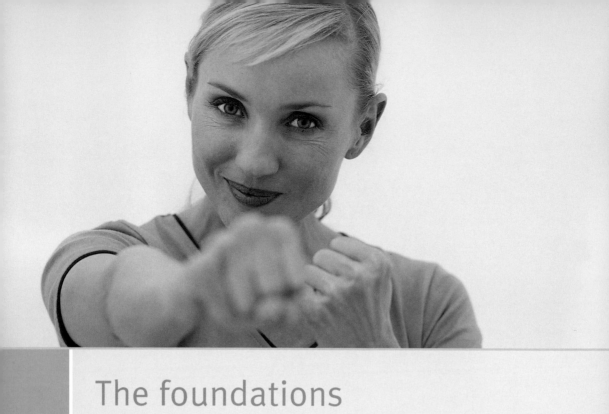

The foundations of your fitness

A tailor-made, varied training program – what does that actually mean? What are the foundations for an effective program that will benefit your figure and your health?

Your personal fitness is defined most of all by four factors that are closely related: strength and stamina, mobility and coordination.

At the heart of the matter is the strengthening of all of your muscle groups, together with exercises which serve to improve or maintain your mobility.

Stamina training forms the basis of your capacity for exercise. You will also benefit from this in the workouts found in the practice section of this book.

Coordination is the fun element of training. Well-developed coordination will give you flowing, harmonious movement. It also reduces the risk of injury as well as the load on your joints when training.

The weekly training plans at the end of the book will show you examples for the best way to build your very own weekly fitness program.

WHAT GOOD FITNESS STUDIOS HAVE TO OFFER

Renowned fitness expert Maria Ljungqvist (41) develops new fitness programs for ELIXIA Health and Wellness Group and ensures the highest quality standards for their 52 fitness and wellness clubs in Germany and Europe. The company represents a holistic approach to fitness with its "ELIXIA-Way" philosophy.

How can a fitness studio supplement your at-home training?

A studio can support your decision to train with professional advice, guidance and a suitable training plan. Particularly at the beginning, many women face the problem of overcoming their own weakness and just getting started. A training program at home, supplemented by a group class, swimming or sauna in a fitness club, can really help you to reach your goals and improve your quality of life.

What additional benefits can fitness clubs offer to women over 40?

In good fitness studios individual exercise programs are created that also take into account health problems; there's sports health advice and also lots of classes for people over 40 – gentler, lower impact that take "problem areas" into account such as the back or joints. Such classes include yoga, classic fitness training, Pilates and of course all water-based classes which are particularly gentle on the joints as well as being effective.

What is the difference in your clubs between a program for women over 40 and classes for younger people?

The level is increased more slowly in order to avoid unhealthy strains. For correct cardiovascular exercise after 40, it is important when exercising in the aerobic zone to remain at up to about 75 percent of the maximum heart rate. Our fitness clubs offer, for example, check-ups upon registration and you can rent pulse-monitor watches for your training. A combination of strength and stamina training as well as relaxation is recommended. Walking, power-walking and cycling strengthen the cardiovascular system; targeted strength training on equipment strengthens the musculature. Our guests can relax in the wellness zone with a steam bath, bio-sauna or massage and in Body & Mind orientated workouts such as yoga.

Strength

The exercise instructions in most fitness books do not differentiate between men and women and are orientated on the whole towards the physiology and constitution of men. But since the muscles of the female body have different requirements in exercise, the recommendations for men often miss the mark for women. The training concept put forward in this book rests on the most up-to-date scientific knowledge about what is most important for women over 40.

Don't worry about developing bulging muscles

Don't worry: even with regular strength training you won't turn into a muscle-bound bodybuilder. This is especially because female hormones under natural conditions will simply not allow such extreme muscle growth. You will soon find this out for yourself. With a balanced exercise program your body will not grow in size but will often even decrease. There is also no point in doing strength training at maximum capacity over a long period, since the female musculature is only designed to increase in size over a relatively short timeframe. The sex hormone testosterone, which is much less available to women than to

men, is mainly responsible for this. If a muscle is slack through lack of exercise or even wasted due to long-term disuse, exercise will first of all add mass. But if the muscle was already being regularly worked before, then it will become firmer and stronger in women, but not bigger.

So don't set yourself the goal of becoming as strong as an ox, but be happy with shapely, strong and sleek muscles. For your workout practice, this means that you should increase the number of repetitions gradually and not overtax yourself.

Focus on abdomen, back and hip extensor muscles

Different values for men and women don't just apply to muscle girth, different muscle groups also respond particularly well to training.

For women the muscles of the arms, legs and shoulder region in particular are less easily trained, while the muscles of the waist area can be built up just about as easily as they can for men. Therefore the focus of your workout should be less about the limbs; it is much more worthwhile for you to train the muscles of the abdomen, back and buttocks. You have a particular advantage when it comes to exercises which stem from the pelvis – the necessary coordination is especially well-developed in women. So exercises suitable for you include technically demanding gymnastic exercises or exercises with elastic bands or using cable-pulls in the fitness studio.

Strength-stamina training comes first

When working on weight machines in the fitness studio it is recommended that you work in sets of 15 to 25 repetitions. This will improve your strength-stamina rather than your maximum weight strength. This depends on you always selecting weights which are not too heavy for you, because only then can you actually manage the recommended number of repetitions. This has the additional advantages that you will be less likely to injure yourself and you won't strain your body's mechanism (page 10). There will be less strain on your cardio-vascular system too; if you only train just so intensely that you don't overtax yourself, you can let your breath flow easily and rhythmically. Among other things, this prevents your blood pressure from rising too high. With the exercises in this book you are working against your own body weight. So it's best to exercise in sets of between 10 and 15 repetitions. If you do more reps you increase the risk of straining muscles and joints by moving incorrectly. That's why we

recommend fewer repetitions here than when working with machines.

You should also be aware that ...

When exercising the arms and legs you should be particularly aware that the elbows and knees can quickly become overstretched. This is how, for example, women often become "knock-kneed", because of their wider pelvis. Make sure not to load your joints when in an over-stretched position.

Targeted training for your pelvic floor should also be a permanent fixture in your program. It's effective against incontinence problems (bladder weakness) that frequently occur during the years of menopause. You will find special exercises for the pelvic floor on page 108.

However you put together your training program, please always include time for a

HOW TO FIND THE RIGHT FITNESS STUDIO

You can tell a good fitness studio primarily by how much time the members of staff take to comprehensively and competently advise you – for example, about which weights are best for you and the appropriate exercises, equipment and number of repetitions.

TIP

meaningful warm-up and a cool-down to finish (from page 60). After 40 the body needs longer to prepare for hard work and to switch over to recovery mode afterwards.

Stamina

What does stamina training add to Bodystyling? Plenty! For example, a good basic level of stamina ensures that your body can better cope with the stresses of a workout. This means that you are able to move in a much more relaxed manner and at the same time work harder. On top of this is the slimming effect of the stimulation to your metabolism.

Moderate effort

Since it is unfortunately biologically impossible to convert fat directly into muscle (even if the adverts keep telling you it is!), you have to select your activities carefully and perform them at the right level. Stamina sports in particular are especially good for this since they are far and away best suited to working with the metabolism.

What's required is not intense but measured loading such as you get with power-walking or gentle jogging. The important thing is not to end up with a face as red as a beet and racing pulse but to feel comfortable throughout the exercise. You should still be able to carry on a conversation without gasping for breath.

There are also other reasons why you should not overdo your stamina program; at a particular amount and a certain training intensity the risk of disruption of the menstrual cycle increases. This is particularly true for high-level athletes, and around half struggle with these kinds of issues. This is an especially critical problem in top-level sports. If, as a result of excessive exercise, a woman's body-fat level sinks below 12 percent (it is on average 28 percent for women!), then she can expect her period to stop completely.

This problem is less common in swimmers than it is in runners, as the body-fat level tends to drop less drastically in water sports. Fat is important as an insulation layer under the skin when swimming. Extreme stamina training can also lead to a drop in estrogen levels which can lead to osteoporosis over the long term.

Revving up your fat-burning engine

Stimulating the metabolism is especially suitable for women. Genetically, they possess around a third more fat reserves

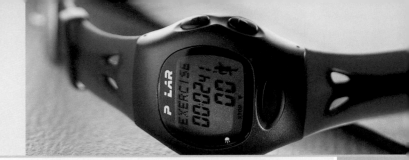

TIP

> Alongside the rule of thumb that you should exercise without getting out of breath, you should also check your pulse from time to time. You can use the following formula as a rough guide. It will roughly give you your maximum pulse rate, i.e. the highest possible number of beats per minute of your heart when exercising: 226 (beats) minus your age per minute.

> If you want to burn fat when exercising you have to stay in a zone between 60 and 70 percent of your maximum value. If your pulse goes much higher you will be burning predominantly carbohydrates instead of burning off those large fat reserves. The great thing about it is that in the fat-burning zone you can continue to exercise for a long time without getting tired.

> Simpler and also more accurate than measuring your pulse at your wrist is to use a heart rate monitor to determine your ideal level of exercise. The monitor consists of a wrist-band pulse monitor and a chest-band (available in sporting goods shops).

than men. But in the spirit of equality and justice they can tap into their fat stores much more easily! This assumes, of course, that they exercise regularly and at the right levels. After about the age of 40, stimulating the metabolism (or fat-burning) is twice as effective. At this time, without stimulation the metabolism gradually changes; muscles increasingly lose mass and fat is more readily stored (see page 20).

Combi-training is best

The best strategy for your figure lies in a combination of one of the stamina sports to stimulate your metabolism and one of the muscle workouts. This way you will enable your whole body to be active for longer periods of time, turbo-boost your fat-burning metabolism and do your whole posture and figure a world of good.

Mobility

Your mobility is what determines how far you can move around in your day-to-day activities and in sports. Particularly for young women, their mobility is very good since women's muscles and tendons are more elastic compared to men. You can keep your mobility for a long time too – if you pursue the correct strategy.

Stay supple!

Loss of mobility tends to appear at around 40, when the muscles and ligaments slowly begin to lose elasticity. You can put an end to these losses – by stretching regularly. This will encourage the harmonious interplay of muscles, ligaments and joints. Your muscles will stay supple and your ligaments and tendons remain elastic – an important requirement if you are to load your joints evenly.

Stretching is especially important if you use particular body parts unevenly in your daily life. If, for example, you sit at a computer a lot you will know all about these problems from experience; the muscles in the hip area, lumbar spine and neck become strained and sore. Gentle stretches – together with strengthening the muscles for better posture – are generally very helpful here. You will find all of the important information about the correct way to stretch and appropriate exercises from page 59 onwards.

Coordination

Try the following experiment: when sitting, place both hands on your knees.

Now grasp your nose with your right hand and with your left hand grasp your right ear. Now place both hands back on your knees and do the movement the other way around. Can you do it repeatedly without a problem? Congratulations! Your coordination is in top condition. If the exercise presents problems for you (as it does for most people), don't give up. Even your coordination can easily be exercised and trained.

A branching "switchboard"

All of your movements are coordinated by a complicated central switchboard – your nervous system. This is the basis for every meaningful movement of your body, for dexterity, your reflexes and a good sense of balance.

Typical woman!
The better your coordination the more supple and elegant, purposeful and precise your movements will be. This is a typically feminine talent, by the way, that you should make use of in your training. If you want to continuously improve your coordination you can, with increasing experience, look for more technically demanding exercises instead of just increasing the number of repetitions or raising the level of difficulty.

Everything in balance

The many varied sports available, particularly those with more demanding technique, offer good opportunities to improve coordination or to maintain it. Activities involving music and dance are very well suited for this since they demand high levels of coordination and are therefore excellent in training it. It is especially important to improve your sense of balance. With good balance you will have a stable stance and be confident in your movements. Stability is extremely important in connection with osteoporosis (see page 18) since a fall would be particularly dangerous with the increased brittleness of the bones.

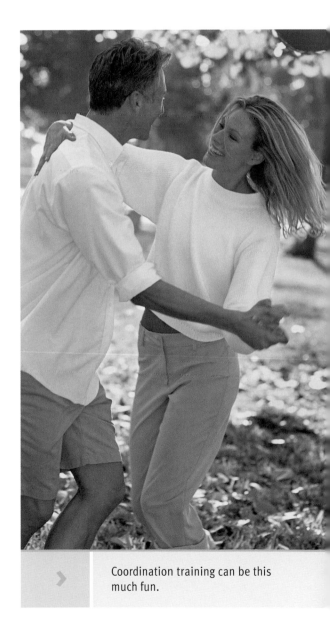

> Coordination training can be this much fun.

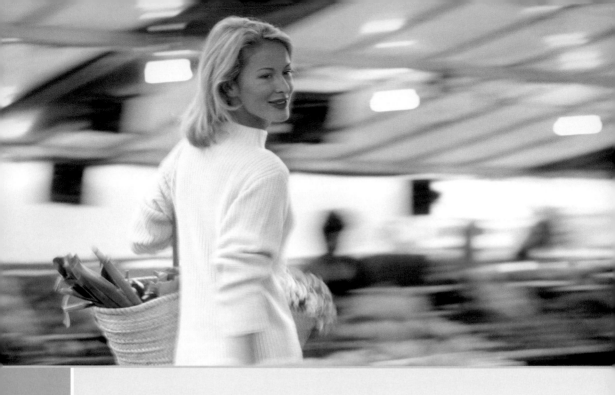

Your bodystyling menu

If you (also) have an issue with weight control, the principle is as simple as it is logical – you will only lose weight if you consume fewer calories than you use. No matter what they promise you in the commercials – there is no miracle product and no clever fitness gadget that will overcome this basic biological principle. After about 40 your body also starts to burn fewer calories. So if you still eat as much as you ever did you will, perhaps, soon begin to be amazed at your new plumper self.

If, though, you simply eat less you will lose muscle mass much more quickly than fat. And if this happens your body will use fewer calories. The result – after your diet you will soon weigh more than before. But don't worry, with regular training and a balanced diet you will easily get back in control of your figure.

Always make sure that you eat all of the important nutrients in sufficient quantities. This is particularly important for your health when you exercise.

The right foods

The following combination has proven an unbeatable recipe for improving both the figure and health: a vitamin and mineral rich diet focusing on carbohydrates and keeping an eye on the fats, with plenty of good protein and a slightly reduced calorie intake.

Carbohydrates (from whole-grain bread or potatoes, perhaps) are the best fuel for your body when exercising. If your body lacks carbs it will turn to its protein reserves and will pull this from your muscle mass.

Essential: Protein and calcium

Your body needs protein to build muscles. Per pound of body weight, you should consume around half a gram of protein per day. If you eat enough fish, meat, poultry, legumes, dairy products and soy products you will not need expensive protein drinks or bars. Dairy products in particular contain lots of calcium as well, and that is good for your bones (page 18).

Metabolic stimulation

Your metabolism will also be trained by controlled stamina training. At rest as well as under load, your body will burn increasingly more fat and fewer carbo-hydrates. Your body's basic burn rate will increase with every pound of extra muscle, around the clock.

An active lifestyle with regular workouts will ensure that you develop a better sense of your own body and only put into it what will do it good. Your metabolism ensures a balanced energy account. This means that it can adapt more flexibly to the nutrients available and will be more forgiving of little caloric slip-ups.

Finding a rhythm

If you always eat at the same times your metabolism will also find its own rhythm. This way your blood sugar levels will remain stable (see page 22). Only exercise 2 to 3 hours after a large meal. Whenever possible, don't eat high-calorie meals in the evenings. Otherwise there will be too much energy available to your body overnight that it does not need. When at rest this excess energy will be particularly easy to store.

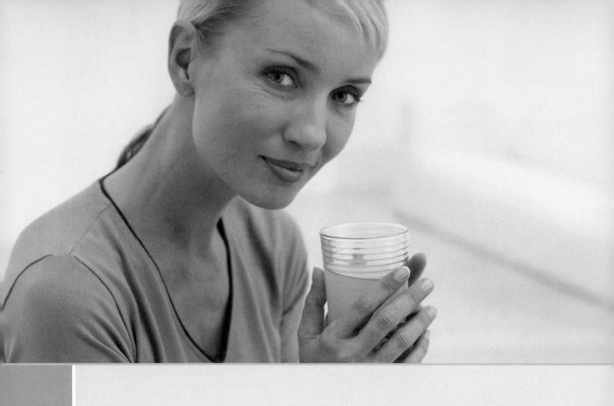

> # Water is life

After oxygen, water is the most important elixir of life. If you drink enough of the right fluids you will stay healthy and able-bodied. Your whole body will be well-supplied with blood and will get enough oxygen and nutrients. Your skin will stay firm and fresh for a long time to come.

But be honest now – are you sure that you are getting enough water to drink? You probably know that adults require around a half gallon of fluids a day. Come on, are you really drinking this much – and is it the right stuff? With the fluid check on page 50 you can work out your "water level" and see exactly how a fluid deficit comes about. Try to at least keep your water account in balance. If you drink more than you need, so much the better; your blood will then be more fluid and can supply the organs all the more effectively. Drinking a lot also has the positive side affect that you will feel less hungry and will consequently eat fewer unnecessary foods that might only put a strain on your body.

Drinking consciously

Take a good look at your drinking habits. Are your favorite drinks also really suited to your body's needs? And do you regularly top off your water tanks so that your body always has enough fluids at its disposal?

Perhaps you have already made the resolution to drink more regularly – you just frequently forget to. Well, simply place mineral water bottles wherever you often spend time, then you'll always be at the watering hole!

The ideal drink

Always reach first for "neutral" drinks such as water, fruit juice and water mixes (water and juice in the ratio 3:1) or tea (herbal, fruit or green teas). This way you'll keep your fluid account in balance and refill your mineral stores after training. Make sure when choosing mineral waters that they contain lots of calcium and magnesium but not very much sodium.

Not suitable as thirst quenchers

Milk does provide fluid, calcium and protein but it also contains calories. You should therefore see it as a healthy food rather than as a thirst-quencher and use it appropriately. Beverages such as coffee, black teas, sugary pop or alcohol have a detrimental effect on your fluid balance because they take water from the body instead of providing it – and it's quite a big gap. If, for example, you drink 8 fluid ounces of cola you will lose about the same amount of fluid from your system.

Staying fluid

The feeling of thirst is nowhere near sufficient to maintain your fluid levels. As a rule you only experience thirst when your body has already lost 16–33 ounces of fluid. So drink regularly and make a habit out of it.

You should bring your intake up to at least 66 fluid ounces per day.

As a rule of thumb, you should drink around 10 glasses (8 fl. oz.) of liquids in small sips spread out over the day. If you take part in sporting activities or generally sweat a lot your needs will be considerably higher.

Ideally, drink during workouts too since your body needs topping off. Only drink small amounts at a time – and slowly! In any case you should replace any fluids lost through sweating immediately after training.

INFO

FLUIDS CHECK

With the help of this table you can roughly work out your actual "water level". Simply fill in the missing values and proceed as in the example below.

Fluid supply		Fluid loss	
Neutral drinks such as mineral water, pure fruit juice and water mix (1/3 juice, 2/3 water), fruit and herbal teas, milk	.... fl. oz.	Elimination by urination and stools; skin and lungs	81 fl. oz.
Fluids in solid foods (in a normal diet, according to amount) 600–900 ml	20–30 fl. oz.	Usage in sport: 8 fl. oz. per 15 mins of sport	.... fl. oz.
Water of metabolism (produced in the body's cells by metabolic process)	10 fl. oz.	Caffeine drinks (e.g. cola or coffee), black tea, alcohol	.... fl. oz.
total supply	.... fl. oz.	total loss	.... fl. oz.

Example: You drink 1 glass of milk (6 fl. oz.), 2 cups of fruit tea (2 x 5 fl. oz.) and a bottle of mineral water (25 fl. oz.). That adds up to 41 fl. oz. of fluid. In addition there are on average 20 fl. oz. which you consume over the day in normal portions of food. Together with the water of metabolism (10 fl. oz.) this adds up to a water intake of 71 fl. oz.

Since the average daily fluid loss in adults due to elimination and the body's basic needs is at least 81 fl. oz. it is already clear that you have insufficient fluid available to you. If you have done half an hour of sport (16 fl. oz.), have drunk a cup of coffee in the afternoon and 1 glass of wine (7 fl. oz.) in the evening, the total loss adds up to 111 fl. oz.. So you are missing 40 fl. oz. of fluid!

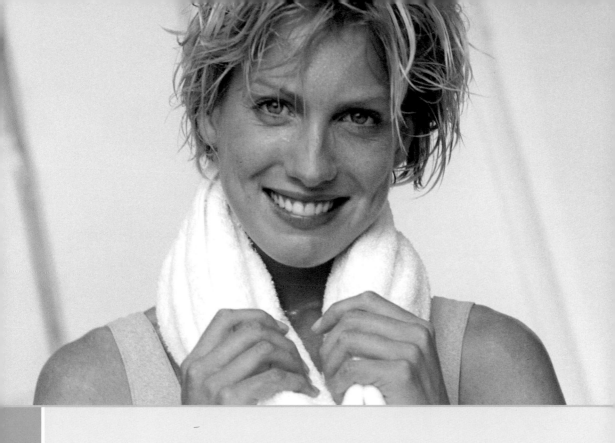

Successful training

Naturally, you want to make your training as effective as possible. No problem! Simply put together a program to suit you, which you can adapt as time goes on. Your body will let you know if you are still training within your personal comfort zone. Sounds easy? It is! On the following pages you will learn how you can create a tailor-made training plan. To get started you just need the right exercises – all of which you can find in this book, starting on page 59. They are the most effective Bodystyling workouts, precisely designed for the needs of women over the age of 40.

Read the tips on the following pages carefully so that your individual exercise program will be a guaranteed "success".

Timing etc.

If your training is to be effective, how often, when and for how long you exercise must play a role. The correct sequence of exercises is also important.

A sensible timetable

Plan to fit your workout into your daily schedule at least 2 to 3 times per week. Spread the exercise units evenly over the week (see Training Plans from page 118).

You can also train more frequently but shouldn't work the same muscles intensely on consecutive days. If you train daily you should divide your workouts up according to focus areas – so concentrate for example on the legs one day, on the arms the next. What time of day you train is up to you. Many people prefer to exercise in the evenings when the body is particularly ready for action and prepared to burn off the energy stored from the day's meals.

If you want to build up your strength as well as your stamina, this is best done on separate days or in separate training sessions. If you want to combine both in one session then stick to the following rule: stamina before strength if you want to focus on burning fat; strength before stamina if you are focused on building your strength.

Success with circuits

If you want to improve your figure in particular, you should give circuit training a try. Here, you move in a circle from one set of exercises to the next. If you are activating certain muscle groups which are remote from each other each time, you can even leave out the breaks between the sets. The number of repetitions is reached by building up several sets of 5–8 repetitions one after the other.

10 minute rounds

For training in "circuits" you can, for example, adapt the 10-Minute Turbo workout on page 115; instead of doing all of the repetitions for each exercise at once and then moving on to the next exercise, change after one complete movement – until you have been through each exercise 10–12 times. Don't include the stretches here but do them as preparation and to conclude the whole session.

With a little experience you can later adapt your own exercise plans to circuits.

Quality is the key!

Always remain completely concentrated during your workouts and don't work until you are completely exhausted.

Measured exercise is much more effective, especially when you have the right technique.

How intensively to train?

New studies have shown that you don't need to push yourself nearly so hard in order to achieve real success. Even a mid-level effort is plenty. And you will protect your circulation as well as muscles, tendons and joints.

Trust your instincts!

End the repetitions when you feel that you would have to stop after the next two or three. After a short break, in which you should drink a little water, you can carry on with the next exercise. Always choose the exercises/variations for which you can manage the recommended number of repetitions. It's a great feeling when you are later able to master even bigger challenges!

The right technique

You should always stabilize your buttocks, stomach and back muscles in the start position – actively tense them. Perform the exercises at a steady pace and without forcing or "bouncing". For abdominal exercises, for example, curl up the upper body within one or two seconds, hold briefly at the furthest

point of the curl, and then uncurl the upper body again with the muscles still tensed, again taking one or two seconds. Go as far as you can go in each of these exercises without pushing the limits of your joints, or even going beyond them. Fit the pace to the rhythm of your breathing. The most taxing part of the exercise should fall on the exhale. Breathe evenly and deeply. So that you don't forget to breathe (correctly), you can breathe in and out so that you hear each breath.

THE RIGHT AMOUNT OF EFFORT

If you feel fit you can do one or two more repetitions than in the book or try the "advanced" variation. The fitness studio staff will know how many repetitions to recommend. Don't overtax yourself; heavy breathing or jittery muscles are clear signs that you are working too hard.

!

IMPORTANT

Four great partners for your workout

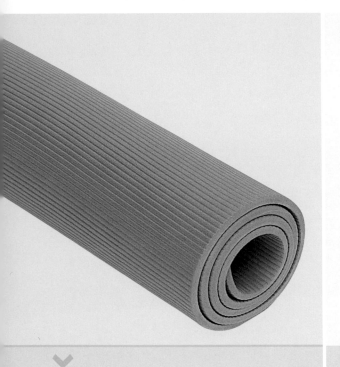

WEIGHTS

For beginners, weights of 2 lbs each (from sporting goods shops) are recommended. Later, you can increase to 4 lbs.
In the beginning, plastic bottles filled with sand or water will also do the trick. However, it is important that you can grasp them firmly.

EXERCISE MAT

Foam exercise mats, which you can find in sporting goods shops, are non-slip and help protect your joints.
You can also use a camping mat or a large folded towel. But beware: Whatever you use should not be able to slip away – check that it will stay put on the floor.

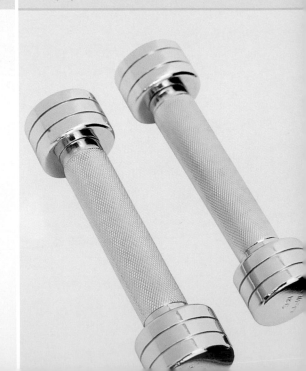

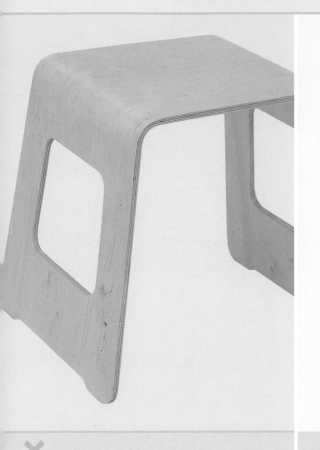

SHOES

Any sports shoe with a firm yet flexible sole is suitable. They should fit you without slipping. If it isn't too cold for you, you can also do many of the exercises barefoot. Wherever you need a good, solid stance, shoes with a grippy sole are recommended.

STOOL

For some exercises you will need a sturdy stool with a flat seat. If it isn't upholstered you can lay your mat or a folded towel on it. A sofa footstool (not too soft) is also good for the job.

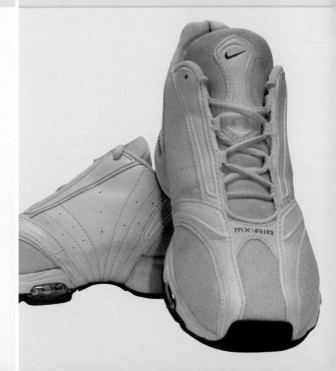

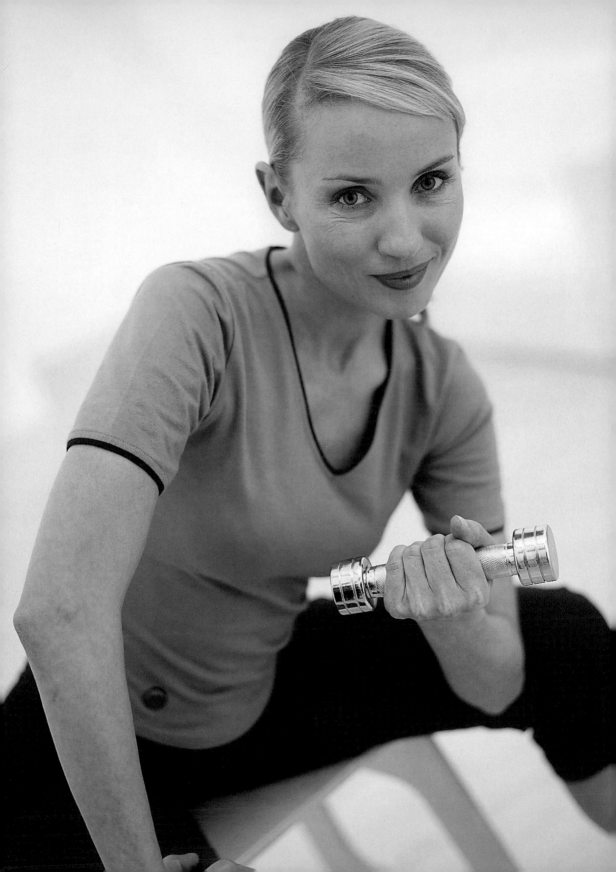

How to get
into top shape

Well-toned muscles, good posture and a
great figure – it's all possible with the right
body sculpting program. After just a few
weeks you will see the results and you will
appear more radiant and confident. The
exercises are so effective that you will have
no problem fitting them in to your schedule.
Get cracking – you won't want to stop!

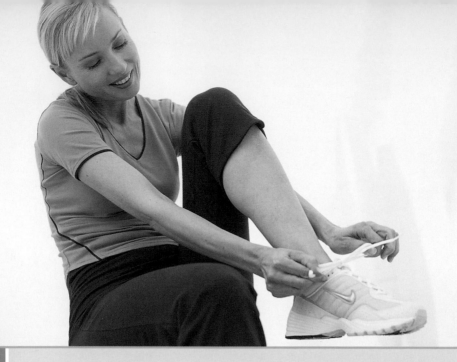

Warm-up and cool-down

Do you start up a cold engine with full revs? Of course you don't – you allow your car the time it needs to warm up. What about your body though – do you always work up gently to full power? Your cardiovascular system and your metabolism also need a few minutes warm-up time in order to adjust to higher demands. The same goes for muscles, tendons, ligaments and joints. So start every training session with the little warm-up and stretching routine on the following pages. It's an investment that will pay back two-fold: You will reduce the danger of over-exertion or even injury on the one hand, and on the other hand you can considerably increase the effects of your exercise. You should also slowly cool down from your training session with stretches (at the end of each segment). Your body will be able to switch more quickly from exertion to rest with this targeted cool-down. So you will feel tired and relaxed in a healthy way instead of feeling restless or even stressed after exercise.

Stretching techniques

Various stretching techniques have
proved themselves useful in exercise,
but they each have their advantages
and disadvantages.

Static stretching

With this technique, you move slowly
and in a controlled manner into a
position in which you feel a definite
stretch but absolutely no pain. Hold this
position for a few seconds and focus on
the muscles that you are currently
stretching. When you notice that the
stretched feeling is dissipating you can
carefully extend the movement slightly
until you feel the original intensity again.
In this way you work up to the stretch
inch by inch and thus improve mobility
over the long term. This method is
excellent for improving your awareness
of your body. The static stretch technique
has another advantage that is particularly
beneficial to beginners: It is almost
impossible to injure yourself using this
method. Static stretching does, however,
reduce the base tension of the muscles.
This is not desirable before sporting
activities in which speed plays an
important role.

Dynamic stretching

In this technique the muscle is stretched
with very gentle bouncing. But the controlled pushing of the stretch has
nothing to do with straining. Here, too,
the stretch must be controlled. Do not
force the muscle and do not load it to the
point of pain or beyond. Otherwise it
can contract protectively and cramp or it
can even result in injury. Advantages of
the dynamic stretching over static
stretching: With the gently bouncing
stretch the muscle loses less of its base
tension which is necessary for quick
movements (for example in sprints);
with dynamic stretching recovery after
sport can also take place more quickly.
You can perform the stretching exercises
in this book as either static or dynamic
according to your needs and experience.

**DON'T STRETCH
FOR TOO LONG!**

Under no circumstances should you
stretch for too long either before or
after a workout. Your muscles will
lose too much of their base
tension. You need this when excercising and in your day-to-day life.
Please stick to the recommended
times given for each exercise.

IMPORTANT

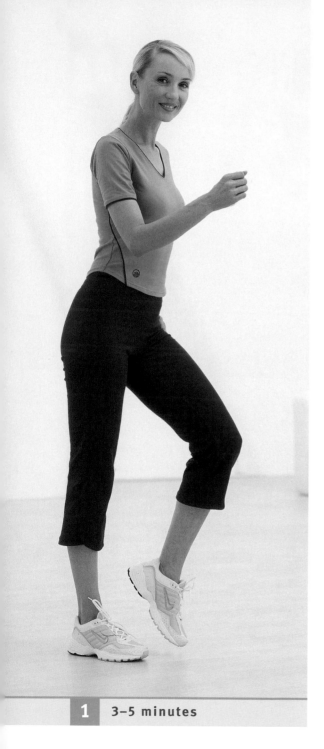

1 | 3–5 minutes

Warm-up

In order to prepare your body for the following workout, begin with the exercise "walking in place". The walking movements will bring your circulation up to speed, loosen up the whole body and ensure good blood flow to the muscles. These are also important requirements for the stretching which follows. You will also become familiar with a few exercises that will prepare important joint and muscle groups for the workout with gentle stretches (so-called mobilisation exercises). This will provide the best foundation for all of the subsequent exercises and protect you from pulled muscles and injuries.

Walking in place

> Stand upright with relaxed knees. The arms should be bent at the elbow at about 90 degrees.
> Now walk gently in place. Bring your knee gently upwards. Always roll the feet forwards from the heel to the ball. Move the opposite arm in time: if you take a "step" with the left leg, the right arm moves forward and vice versa. 1

Preparing the hip joint

> Stand with one leg well in front of the other with knees slightly bent. Lift the heel of the back leg off the floor. Your hands should be on your hips. **2**

> Now move the hips slightly forward. At the same time draw your navel backwards and lightly tense the buttocks. **3** When you feel a stretch in the crook of the hip, hold the position for a few seconds, then go back to the start position.

2   **8 times per side**

3

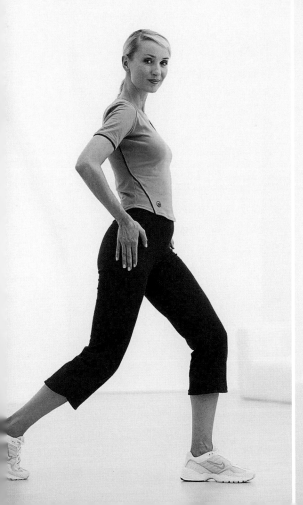

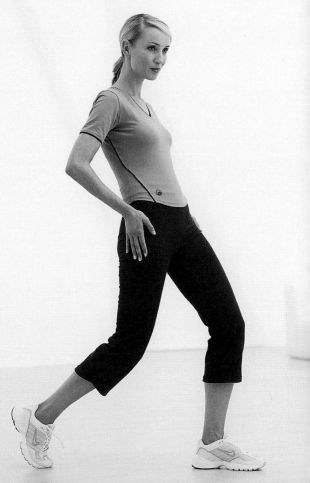

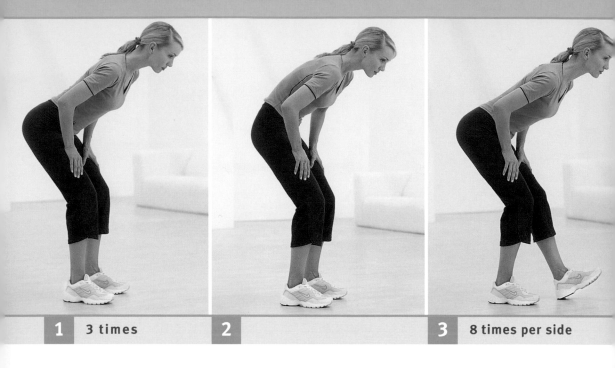

1   3 times   **2**   **3**   8 times per side

Stretching the lower back

> Stand with legs hip-width apart and knees slightly bent. Support your hands on your thighs and keep your back straight. Look towards the floor so that your neck remains completely relaxed. **1**
> Now curve your lower back by drawing your navel up towards the ceiling. Make sure that only your lower back moves. Shoulders, head and legs stay still. Hold the stretch for a short time. **2**
> Straighten the back once more.

Preparing the backs of the thighs

> Stand with legs hip-width apart. Your left foot should be about one foot-length in front of your right.
> Support your hands on your thighs and, with a straight back and shoulder blades slightly drawn together, bend the right leg; at the same time push your buttocks backwards. The left leg remains stretched out. **3**
> Now move slightly lower with your upper body by pushing your chest and buttocks towards the floor until you feel a light stretch in the back of the thigh. **4**
> Relax.

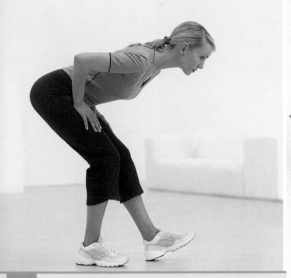

4

Stretching the chest muscles

> Stand with your legs about shoulder-
  width apart and the toes and knees
  pointing slightly outward. Stretch the
  arms out to the sides at about
  shoulder height. The palms should be
  facing up towards the ceiling.
> Now push the arms slowly further
  backwards until you feel a stretch in
  the area of the chest muscles. 5
> Bring the arms back to the start
  position.

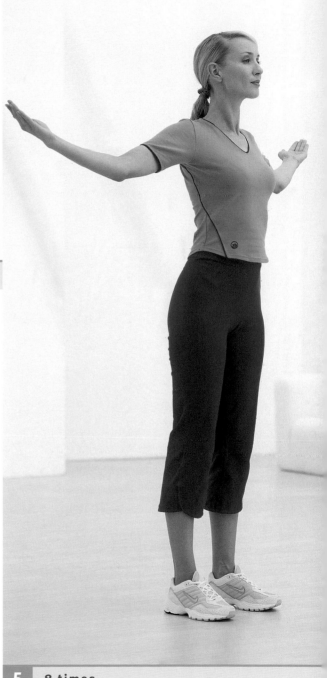

5 8 times

Cool-down

Here are some ideas on how you can leave your workout feeling totally relaxed. On the right you will find more tips for the relaxation phase.

All-around relaxation

You need a large, thick cushion (or several smaller ones) which you should place on the floor or training mat.

> Lie on your back and place your calves on the cushion(s). The arms lie relaxed alongside the body. Your head should be totally relaxed, so pull your chin slightly towards your chest. You can

also put a flat cushion beneath your head.

> Close your eyes and breathe deeply into your abdomen; then let the air flow out again. Feel the sensation of deep relaxation flowing through your whole body. Notice how your loose, well-oxygenated muscles now feel.

> After a few minutes you can very slowly and gently turn your head alternately to left and right to finish.

An "extra round" of relaxation ...

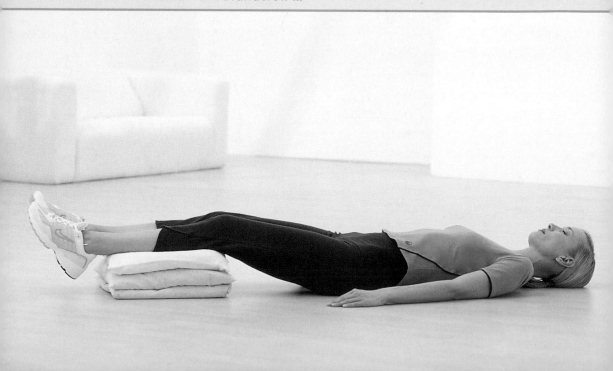

RELAXING AND STRETCHING: FOR A WELL-BALANCED WORKOUT

› HELP YOUR BODY TO SWITCH OVER

Whatever happens, allow yourself to complete the suggested exercises for relaxation and regeneration at the end of each session. Your body needs time to recover from the demands of exercise and your mind will also switch over more easily from activity to recovery. Gentle stretching stimulates the regenerative processes of the body, ensures clear thoughts and gives you renewed vigor.

› AN ACTIVE BREAK FOR THE METABOLISM

Within a measured cool-down period the body can recover from the demands of exercise and regenerate more effectively. Your metabolism has got a lot to do at the moment: Surplus substances which have built up in your body during your workout must be carried away and depleted reserves must be replaced.

› RELEASING TENSION

Loosen up your entire musculature again directly after your workout. You can do this, for example, by shaking out your arms and legs or by swinging them gently back and forth. In addition, muscles that have been particularly stressed during exercise should be carefully stretched with the appropriate movements. That way tight muscles are loosened up again before it comes to unpleasant aches and pains.

› WITH STRETCHING THE EMPHASIS IS ON "GENTLY"

Muscles that have been stressed and are therefore tired due to exercise are particularly sensitive to stretching. Therefore you should always practice the stretches gently. This is especially true for the gently bouncing stretches (see page 59), which have the advantage over static exercises in that they support regeneration more effectively.

› PLANNED RELAXATION

In the practice section of this book you will find the right stretches for every muscle group. In the weekly training plan and in the 10-minute workout at the end of the book you can find the recommended cool-down exercises for each. In addition to the stretches, when you have exercised in the evening, you can do the relaxation exercises on page 64 and allow your body and mind to change gears completely to rest and relaxation.

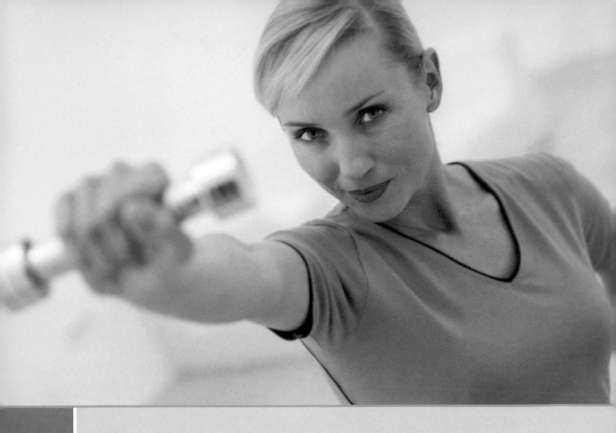

Workout for the upper body

Is upper body exercise nowhere near the top of your list of important things to do? Then you have something in common with the majority of women! But you can improve your posture and protect your back and neck from painful strains with a targeted upper-body workout. The exercises offer a balance to the one-sided stresses of everyday life that particularly affect these body parts.

Last but not least, your confidence will profit from a strong, straight upper body; you will simply be able to go through life more upright and with more pride!

By the way, you shouldn't be afraid of developing masses of muscles – an upper body which has been exercised in a well-balanced way definitely looks graceful and your improved tone will enhance your femininity.

Muscle groups of the upper body

Upper back

The most important area in exercising the upper body is the upper back. Many people often adopt a posture in which the shoulders roll forward. Free your back from this unhealthy position and emphasize your personal radiance with an "unbending posture". The rotators are especially important for this. This is the name for the muscles that pull the shoulders back and thus straighten up the whole upper body.

When you put together your individual training plan you should do two or three exercises for the upper back to every one exercise for the chest muscles in the same exercise unit.

The chest muscles

Perhaps you have heard that exercising the chest muscles makes a small bust more voluptuous. Wrong: With intensive exercising the opposite usually happens. The bust consists mostly of connective and fatty tissue which can get smaller with intensive exercise. But don't worry: this is only a problem for professional sportswomen and weightlifters. It is much more common that proportionate exercise of the large and small chest muscles has a very positive effect. Together with the shoulder muscles, the chest muscles provide support and lift for your bust. A strong back musculature also contributes here, pulling the shoulders back and thus straightening the whole upper body.

Shoulder area

Good shoulders are the result of a well-exercised deltoid muscle. It is involved in all movement of the shoulder girdle. It is important here, aside from a careful warm-up and cool-down, to perform the exercises correctly. Otherwise strains can develop quite quickly in the neck region. You should also stretch your neck from time to time throughout the day.

Arm muscles

They are real head-turners, particularly in the summer – nicely shaped arms with sleek muscle tone. The muscles under the arms, the triceps, are some of the first to lose strength and shape in women over 40. Regular exercise tones the muscles and also keeps the skin tight and smooth.

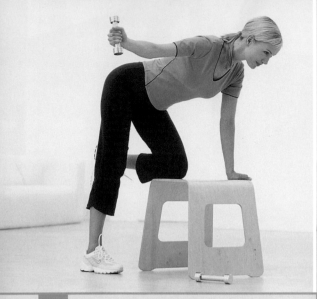

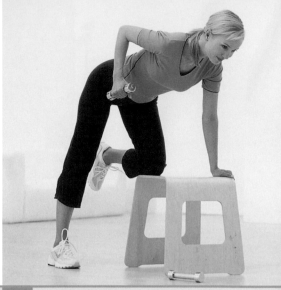

1 | **12 times per side** | **2 sets**

2 | **12 times per side** | **2 sets**

Upper back

Rotators with weight

> Support yourself with your left hand and left knee on a stool. The left arm and left thigh should be roughly perpendicular to the floor. Hold a weight in the right hand. Let the arm hang, gently bent.

> Lift the right arm slowly sideways to shoulder height. At the same time push the right shoulder blade in the direction of the spine and turn the thumb towards the ceiling. Hold this position for a short time. **1**

> Now bring your arm slowly back to the start position.

> **Variation:** As a beginner you could perform the exercise without the weight.

Important: Don't allow your back to hollow! Tip your pelvis slightly backwards so that your back remains straight.

Rowing with weight

> Support yourself on the seat of the stool with your left hand and left knee. The left arm and left thigh should be in a perpendicular position. Hold the weight in your right hand. Let your arm hang down.

> Lift your right arm slowly towards the ceiling, bending it at the same time so that the elbow moves upwards. At the same time pull the right shoulder blade in towards the spine. Hold this position for a short time.

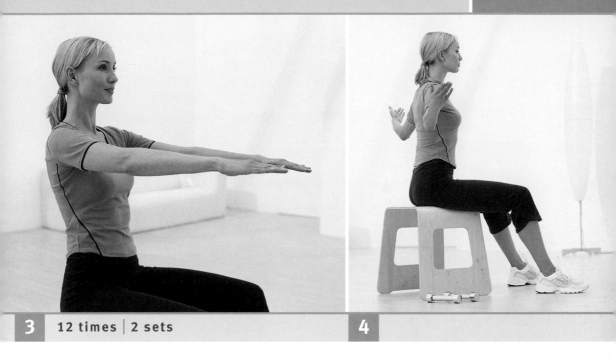

3 12 times | 2 sets   **4**

> Now slowly lower the arm again. Keep the elbow close in to your body while doing so. **2**
> **Advanced:** If you can do the exercise easily, simply hold two weights in your right hand.

Rotators, seated

> Sit on a chair and rest your feet, slightly apart, on the floor. Put your arms out in front of your body so that they are almost straight. Your elbows should be slightly lower than shoulder-height. **3**
> Move the forearms slowly backwards until the elbows are behind the body. Turn your hands so that the thumbs point outwards. Draw the shoulder blades together; keep the shoulders relaxed. Hold this position for a short time. **4**
> Bring the arms slowly back to the start position.

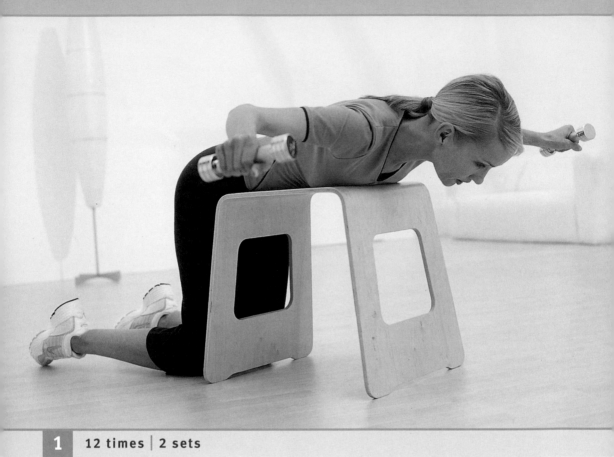

1   **12 times | 2 sets**

Flying on your stomach

> Lie with your stomach on the seat of a stool. Hold a weight in each hand and rest your toes gently on the floor.
> Slowly raise your arms to the sides, to shoulder-height, drawing the shoulder blades together. Hold the position briefly. **1**
> Lower the arms to the start position.
> **Variation:** If you find the exercise too difficult in the beginning, you can also do it without weights.

Apron strings

> Lie on your stomach on a mat. The tips of your toes should be resting on the floor and your buttocks should be gently tensed. Lay your forehead on a folded towel so that your neck is completely relaxed. Stretch your arms above your head and hold them just over the floor. **2**
> Move your bent arms towards your body. The forearms remain pointing forwards. The elbows move towards

the shoulders and then past the shoulders to the torso. **3**

> Turn your arms in so that the palms of your hands face the ceiling and cross your hands over your lower back as if you were tying apron strings. **4**

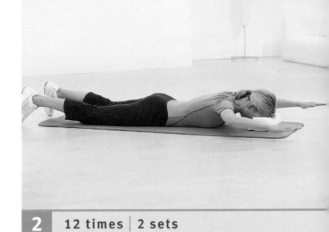

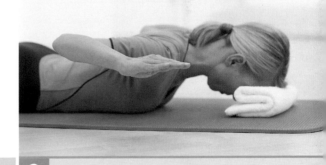

2 | **12 times | 2 sets**

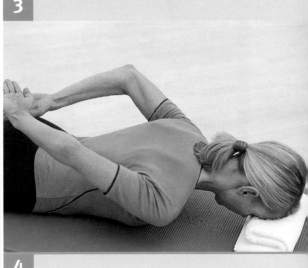

3

4

APRON STRINGS ANY TIME

The apron strings exercise is very effective and you can quickly do a variation in the office: Sit on a chair and raise your arms forward to just below shoulder-height. Now pull your elbows backwards (drawing the shoulder blades together). Now "tie the apron strings" – cross your hands behind your back as in figure 4.

Chest muscles

Pull-over

> Lie with your back on a stool. Place your feet on the floor and lift your buttocks. Grasp a weight with both hands.
> Now lift the weight upwards with almost straight arms until your hands are above your chest. **1**
> Move your arms slowly over your head until the forearms are almost next to your ears. Hold this position for a few seconds. **2**

> Now bring your arms back to the position above your chest.
> **Advanced:** If, after a time, you can easily perform the required number of repetitions, try the exercise with more weight.

1   **12 times | 2 sets**   **2**

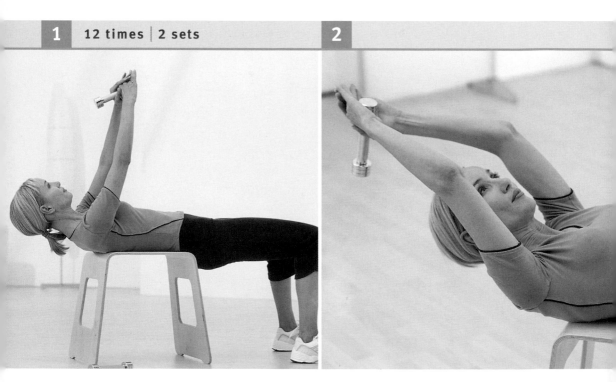

Flying on your back

> Lie with your back on a stool. Place your feet on the floor and lift your buttocks. Take a weight in each hand.
> Now raise your almost straight arms out to the sides and upwards until your hands are above your chest.
> Slowly lower your arms outwards again, keeping your elbows gently bent. Hold briefly when your arms are almost horizontal. **4**
> Now slowly raise them again.

> **Variation:** If the exercise is too difficult for you with weights you can leave them out to begin with. If, later, you can do it with weights you will be able to see the results of your training!

3 12 times | 2 sets

4

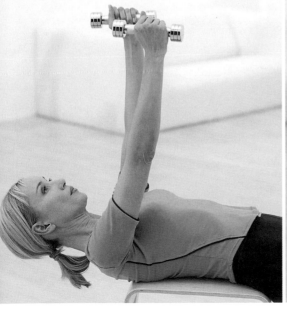

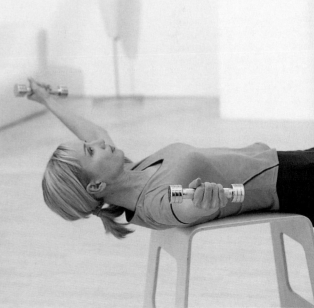

Push-ups

With push-ups you can choose from three different levels depending on your level of fitness. Start with the easiest exercise: push-ups with stool. If you can manage 12 repetitions or more with no problem then congratulations! You can go right away and try the next level.
Important: With all push-ups your stomach should be gently tensed. But don't forget to breathe evenly! Keep the elbows gently bent in order not to strain the elbow joint unnecessarily.

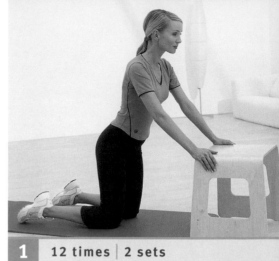

1   12 times │ 2 sets

Easy push-ups

> Lay your mat in front of a stool and support your hands on either side of the seat. The thumbs should point forward. The feet can either rest lightly

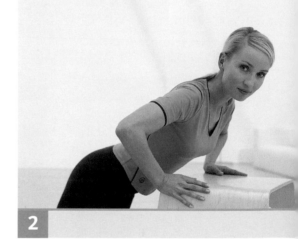

2

PROTECTING THE KNEES

If you want to take the strain off your knees even more, roll up your exercise mat as a cushion for your knees.

on the floor or be lifted off the floor. Gently tense your stomach muscles. **1**
> Now slowly bend your arms until your upper body is almost touching the stool. **2**
> Slowly push upwards again.

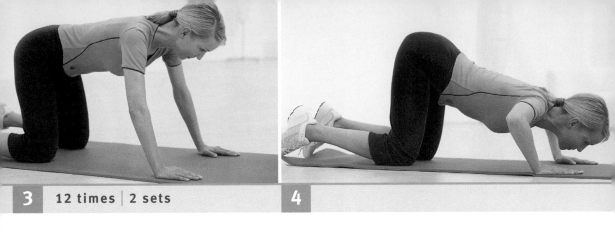

3   12 times | 2 sets   **4**

Medium push-ups

> Kneel on the mat and support your-
self on your hands. The knees should
be directly below the hip joints, the
hands a little more than shoulder-
width apart. The feet should rest
gently on the mat or be slightly lifted
off the floor. Gently tense your
stomach muscles. **3**
> Now slowly bend your arms to lower
your chest. Stop just before you reach
the floor. **4**
> Now slowly go back up to the start
position.

Hard push-ups

> Kneel on the mat, supporting yourself
on your hands. Walk your hands forwards until your upper body forms a
straight line with your thighs. The feet
can rest gently on the floor or be
slightly lifted. Now gently tense your
stomach muscles. **5**
> As in the previous exercise, now
slowly bend your arms so that your
upper body is lowered almost to the
floor. **6**
> Then slowly come back up to the start
position.

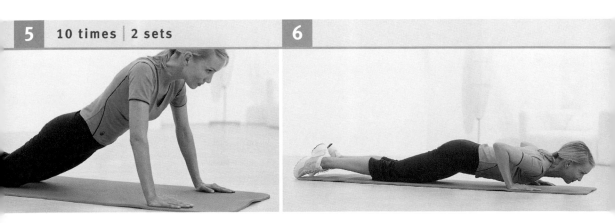

5   10 times | 2 sets   **6**

Shoulders

Side arm raises

> Take a weight in each hand. Stand with your feet slightly more than shoulder-width apart. Your knees and toes should point slightly outwards. Bend the knees slightly and let the arms hang down, slightly bent. Make sure that your upper body is upright.
> Raise the arms to no more than shoulder-height. Don't raise your shoulders. **1**

Forward arm raises, alternate

> Take a weight in each hand. Stand in a walking position; let your arms hang down, slightly bent. The upper body should be upright.
> Raise your straight right arm up slowly in front of you to no more than shoulder height. Do not raise the shoulders. **2**
> Now slowly lower the arm again and repeat the exercise with the left arm.

Overhead press

> Take a weight in each hand. Stand in a walking position and raise the bent

1   10 times | 2 sets   **2**   10 times | 2 sets

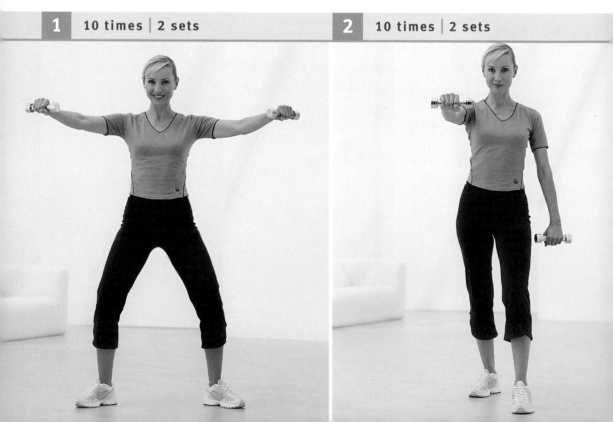

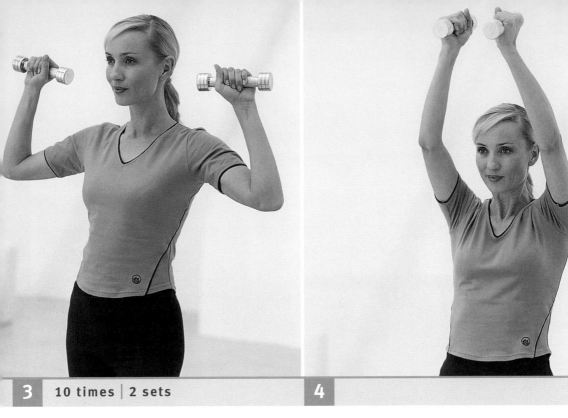

3 10 times | 2 sets

4

arms until the hands are approximately at shoulder height. Your fists should be pointing upwards. **3**

> Now slowly raise your fists further upwards. The fingers of both hands should move towards each other until they are almost touching above your head. Do not raise your shoulders. **4**

> **Variation:** If your neck area is very tense, do the exercise without weights to start with. After a few sessions you can then add the weights.

POWER TO THE SHOULDERS – FAST

Do something every day for your shoulders, at any time. Stand in a door frame. Now place the backs of your hands on the door frame and try to push your arms outwards against the resistance of the frame. Maintain this tension for around 10 seconds then release. You can easily repeat this 3–5 times.

TIP

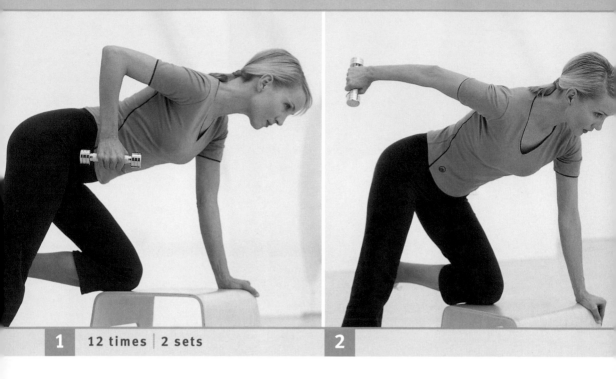

1 12 times | 2 sets

2

Arms

Triceps: Arm stretches

> Stand in front of a stool. Support
> yourself with your left hand and left
> knee on the seat. Hold a weight in
> your right hand. Bend the right arm so
> that the elbow moves back and up. **1**
> Now stretch the right forearm slowly
> backwards. The upper arm should not
> move. Hold the stretch briefly. **2**
> Slowly bend the arm again.
> **Important:** Make sure that the back
> remains straight in order not to strain
> your spine unnecessarily.

Easy dips

> Sit on a stool so that your buttocks
> are right at the front edge of the seat.
> Your lower legs should be perpendicu-
> lar to the floor. Support yourself with
> both hands on the edge of the seat.
> The hands should be pointing
> forwards. Now slide a little further
> forwards until your buttocks are no
> longer touching the seat. **3**
> Slowly bend your arms; keeping the
> elbows pointing backwards. Your
> buttocks should move towards the
> floor and your upper body should

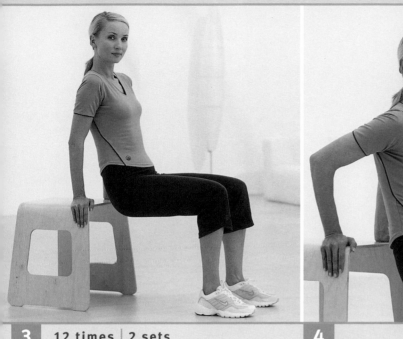
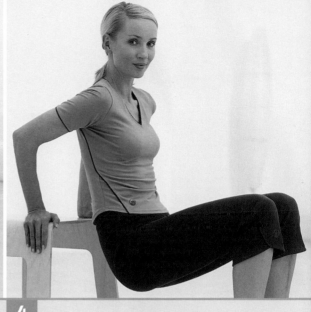

3 12 times | 2 sets   **4**

move slowly downwards past the edge of the stool. Stop when your elbows are about at shoulder height. **4**

> Now slowly push your upper body back upwards. The movement is complete when your elbow joints are still very slightly bent.

DIPS FOR THE OFFICE

You can also exercise your triceps with dips at your desk. The movement is the same as in "easy dips" but now instead of using a stool your desk can really make itself useful for once. Support yourself on your hands on the desk. Now slowly allow your body to sink downward as described in the exercise, and then raise it up again.

TIP

79

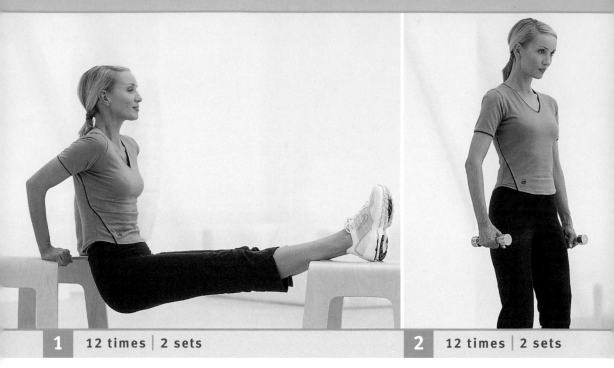

1 12 times | 2 sets

2 12 times | 2 sets

Hard dips

> Place two stools or chairs about 3 feet apart, the seats facing each other. Sit on one stool and lay your feet on the other. Slide your buttocks forward until you are sitting on the edge of the seat. Place your hands, fingers pointing forwards, on the edge of the seat. Slide slightly further forward until your buttocks are no longer touching the seat.
> Slowly bend your arms, the elbows pointing backwards. Your buttocks should move towards the floor, your upper body should slide slowly downwards alongside the edge of the seat. Stop when your elbows are almost at shoulder height. **1**

> Slowly push upwards again. The movement is complete when there is still a very slight bend in the elbow joints.

Biceps: Hammer curls

> Stand with your feet about shoulder-width apart with a weight in each hand. Hold your elbows so that the tips of your thumbs point forward. **2**
> Slowly bend your arms, bringing the forearms upward. At the same time, turn your hands until the backs of your hands point forward. The upper arms should not move. **3**
> Now slowly lower the arms again to the start position.

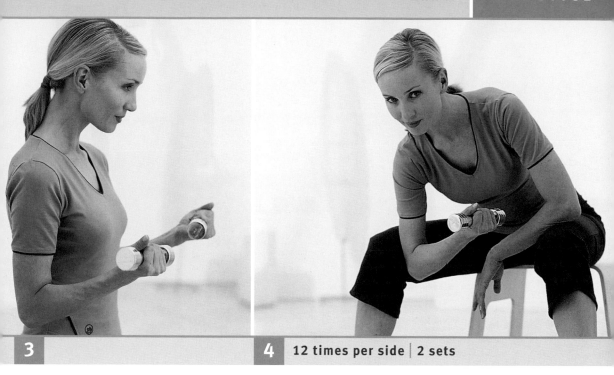

3

4 | **12 times per side** | **2 sets**

Important: Keep your upper body straight, do not lean backwards. If the exercise becomes too much of a strain it is better to take a break.

Biceps curl, one-sided

> Sit on a stool so that your feet are placed firmly on the floor. Hold a weight in your right hand. Support yourself with your left arm on your left thigh. Lean your upper body forward slightly, so that your outstretched right arm moves downwards between your thighs until your right elbow is resting on the inside of your right thigh.

> Now slowly bend your right arm and lift the weight. Hold this position briefly. **4**
> Slowly return the arm to the stretch.
> **Advanced:** If you can easily manage 12 repetitions three times, you can add a second weight to the same hand.

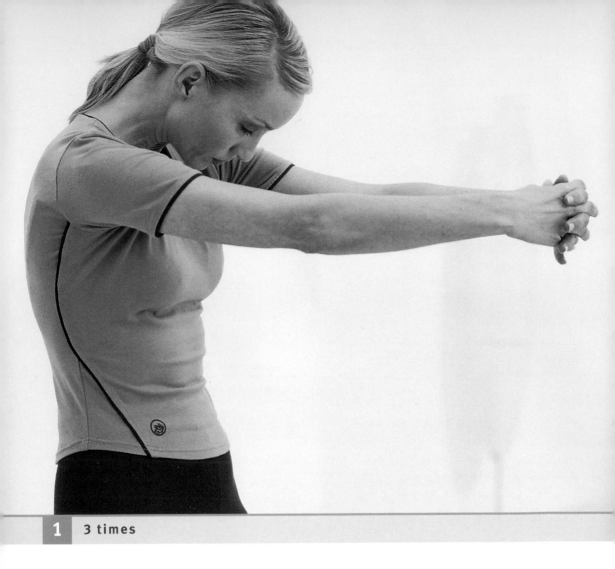

Stretching and relaxing

Upper back

> Stand with legs hip-width apart. Hold your hands clasped in front of your chest.
> Now push your hands and upper body as far forward as you can. At the same time, push your shoulder blades apart and round your upper back until your head is between your arms. 1
> Hold the stretch for about 15 seconds, then slowly release and let your arms hang down.

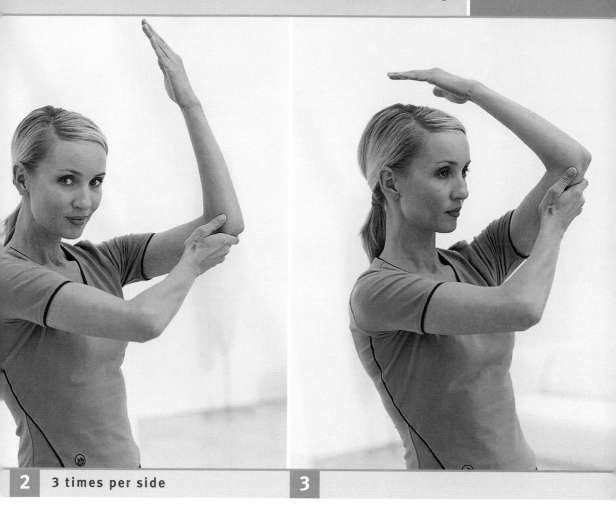

2 3 times per side

3

Triceps

> Stand with legs not quite shoulder-width apart. The toes and knees should point slightly outwards, the legs should be slightly bent. Lift your bent left arm forward until the left elbow is at about shoulder height. Now place your right hand on your left elbow. **2**

> With your right hand, push your left arm upwards. The right upper arm should move towards your head until you feel a stretch in the back of your upper arm. **3**

> Hold the stretch for around 15 seconds, then lower your arms in front of your chest.

Neck

> Stand with your legs hip-width apart and let your arms hang loosely down.
> Lower your head slowly to the right and at the same time pull your left shoulder downwards until you feel a stretch on the left side of your neck. **1**
> Hold briefly, then straighten the head again and relax the shoulder. Now stretch the other side.
> **Advanced:** To increase the stretch, take your right arm behind your body and pull the left arm downwards. **2**
> When you relax the stretch let the arms go.

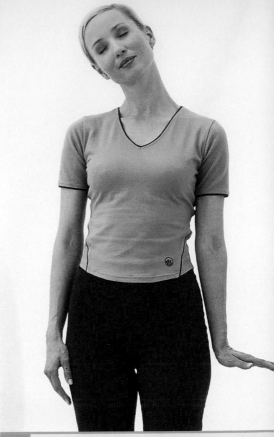

1   3 times

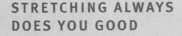

TIP

STRETCHING ALWAYS DOES YOU GOOD

The neck stretch as described above is of benefit anywhere and at any time. It is especially helpful to do it every now and then at your desk or when you make a stop for gas. It can prevent or relieve neck strain and the headaches which it causes.

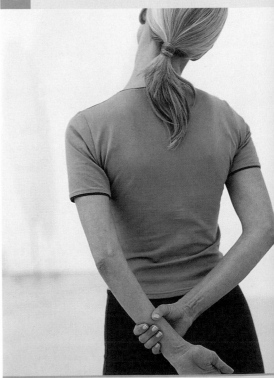

2

Chest stretch I

> Stand with your legs slightly more than shoulder-width apart. The toes and knees should point slightly outwards, the legs should be slightly bent. Loosely bend your arms. Lift them to the sides with the palms facing upwards until your elbows are at around shoulder height.
> Now pull both arms backwards so that you open your chest. **3**
> Hold the stretch for around 15 seconds, then relax. Don't lower your arms between repetitions.

Chest stretch II

> Stand with your legs slightly more than shoulder-width apart. The toes and knees should point slightly outwards, the legs should be slightly bent. Let your arms hang loosely down with the palms facing backwards. Now place one hand on top of the other behind your back.
> Stretch both arms backwards. At the same pull your chin slightly in. **4**
> Hold the stretch for around 15 seconds then slowly relax and lower the arms again.

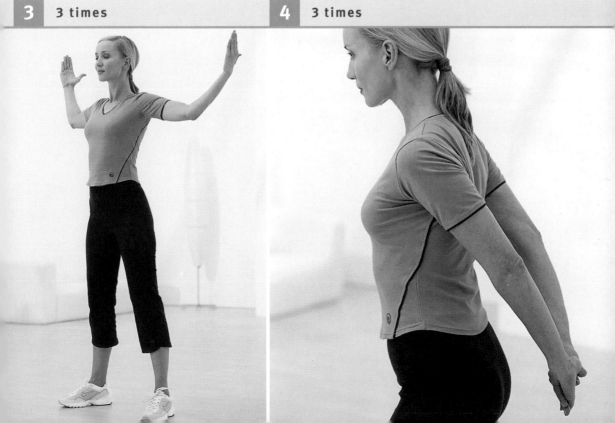

3 3 times   **4** 3 times

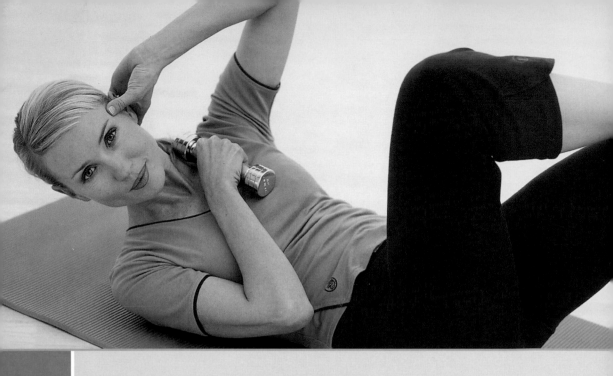

Workout for the mid-section

One of the most important areas to exercise is the abdominal region, and not just because every woman wants to have a nice flat stomach. This region is also home to an area that encounters the most problems in everyday life: the lower back.

Exercises for the abdominal region are known as core-strength training. A well-trained mid-section is very important for your posture and also helps you avoid or rectify back problems. Exercise your abdominal area in every workout. And don't forget to do the stretches afterwards!

Muscle groups of the abdominal area

At the core: Stomach muscles

A flat stomach with well-defined muscles is a sign of fitness and athleticism. And with good reason: the stomach muscles in particular only become visible with regular exercise and after getting rid of the layer of fat across the abdomen. Frequently sitting for long periods of time, however, can weaken the stomach muscles. To redress this imbalance you need targeted exercise.

Basically there are three sections of the abdominal muscles which have three different functions:

The rectus abdominus

They are used in "sitting up" from a supine (lying down) position and in curling up the torso. They serve to stabilize the pelvis, for example when you go up or down a sloped surface. The rectus abdominus holds the pelvis upright and ensures a healthy movement in the lumbar region of the spine.

The obliques

These muscles support the functions of the rectus abdominus. Apart from this, they also come into play when the torso is turned to the side and, together with the diaphragm and the pelvic floor muscles, are responsible for the so-called stomach-press. This plays an important role in lifting heavy loads and in emptying the bladder and the bowels.

The transverse abdominals

They are similarly involved in the stomach-press, hold the waist in shape and help stabilize the spine.
The stomach muscle exercises from page 90 onwards provide all-around exercise for this muscle group.
When excercising the muscles of your mid-section pay particular attention to regular breathing. It is quite easy with these exercises that you may forget to breathe properly!
During the exercises in which the upper body is curled up, try to especially concentrate on the "un-curling".
Always perform the exercises very slowly and don't use force. It is better to do one or two fewer repetitions but to focus on concentrated movements.

Always busy: The lower back

The strains of everyday life put a particular load on your lower back; the consequences of incorrect sitting posture or of lifting improperly may painfully announce themselves in the region of the lumbar spine. In order to take the strain off the back the musculature must be strengthened – poor posture habits will then become a thing of the past.
Always perform the exercises for the lower back muscles very slowly and with small rather than expansive movements.

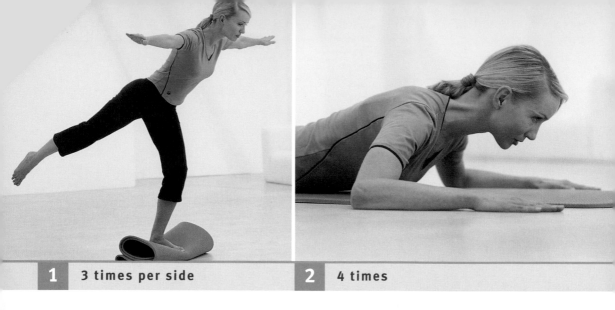

1 3 times per side   **2** 4 times

General strengthening of the mid-section

Balance

> Fold a towel or mat together so that it provides a soft surface. Stand on it, preferably barefoot. Now move your right leg slightly backwards so that you are only supporting yourself with the tips of your toes. The left leg should be slightly bent at the knee. Both arms should be loosely lifted out to the sides.
> Now raise the right foot slightly off the floor. When you have a secure stance, lean your upper body slightly forward. This will bring the right foot further off the floor. Hold this position for a short time. **1**
> Now slowly lower the right leg so that the upper body returns to an upright position.
> **Advanced:** The softer the surface, the more difficult the exercise.

Shoulder push-up

> Lie on your stomach on your mat. Keep looking at the floor. Rest your arms, bent, close to your body so that your elbows are just below shoulder height.
> Now perform the movements in the order specified (!): pull in your navel so that the stomach is lifted slightly from the floor; now draw the shoulders down in the direction of your buttocks; finally, press your lower arms into the floor so that the upper body is raised off the floor. **2**
> Hold the position for about 10 seconds then slowly lower your upper body to the mat once more.

Important: Keep your navel pulled in throughout the entire exercise!

Long support

> Lie with your stomach on the mat. Your toes should be resting on the floor. Place your elbows underneath your shoulders and push the upper body up off the floor. At the same time draw your shoulder blades together.

> Tense your abdominal muscles and draw the navel inwards. Hold this tension and raise your hips off the floor so
that only your knees and toes are supporting your lower body.

> Now also take your knees off the floor and lift your buttocks in the direction of the ceiling. Hold this position for a short time. **3**

> Lower your buttocks to the right until it is just above the floor, "rolling" over your feet to the side. Hold briefly here. **4**

> Now lift your buttocks back to the middle and move them over to the other side. Then come back to the middle again and then lower yourself back to the floor.

> **Advanced:** When you have mastered this exercise you can repeat the rolling to left and right several times before finally lowering yourself back to the floor.

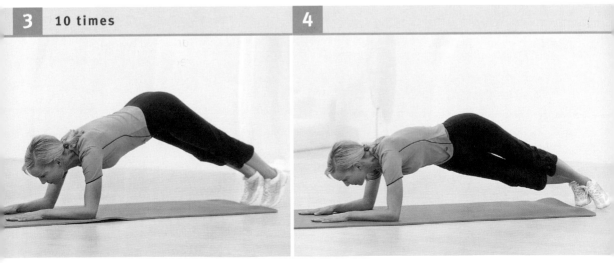

3   **10 times**   **4**

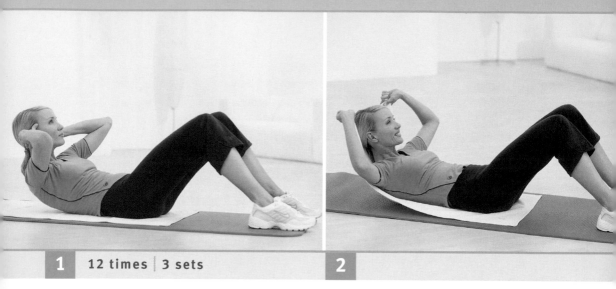

1 12 times | 3 sets   **2**

Stomach and waist

Basic crunch

> Lie with your back on the mat. Place your feet about hip-width apart. Place both hands behind your head with the thumbs on your cheek bones or temples so that your elbows remain pointing outward.

> Slowly raise your upper body until both shoulder blades are lifted off the floor. Hold your head so that you place your fist between your chin and chest. **1**

> Hold this position for around 2 seconds then slowly lower your upper body until your head is just above the floor.

> **Variation:** If you have frequent neck problems or have problems during the exercise, try the following variation: Place a towel behind your head and lift yourself up while holding onto the corners of the towel to the left and right of your head. **2**
This way your head will remain relaxed during the exercise and the pressure will be taken off your neck.

> **Advanced:** The exercise is harder if you perform the movement even more slowly.

> Another possibility for making the exercise harder: Place a weight under your neck and grasp it from above with both hands.

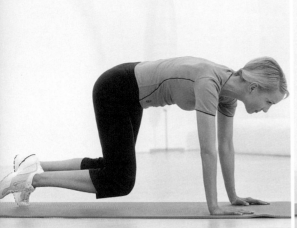
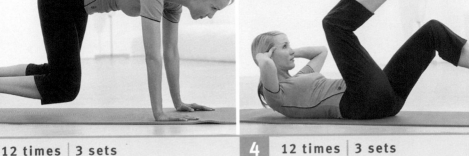

3 12 times | 3 sets

4 12 times | 3 sets

Knee crunch

> Kneel on all fours on the mat. Your arms and thighs should be vertical to the floor. Touch your toes to the floor and lift your knees from the floor so that your thighs and upper body form a right angle.

> Lower your right knee slowly to the floor. **3**

> Lift the knee again and now lower your left knee.

> **Advanced:** The exercise is made more difficult if you support yourself on your forearms and pull your knees alternately in towards your upper torso.

Leg dips

> Lie with your back on the mat. Place your hands under your head. Pull both thighs in toward your upper body.

> Raise your upper body a little. Hold this basic level of tension and slowly lower your bent left leg forward and downward until the heel is just above the floor. **4**

> Then slowly pull the leg in again to the body. Now lower and raise the right leg in the same way.

> **Advanced:** The exercise is made more difficult if you stretch the leg out forward until it is just above the floor.

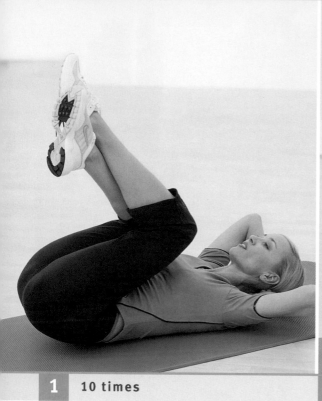

1 10 times

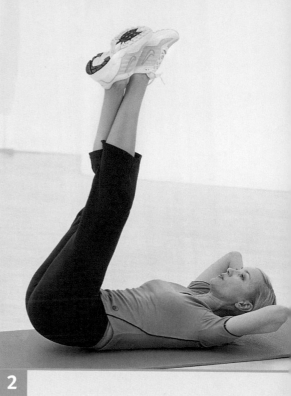

2

Pelvic roll

> Lie on your back on the mat, your head resting in your hands. Stretch your legs, parallel, upward. The knees should remain gently bent. Now cross your ankles.

> Now pull your legs in toward your upper body. Your buttocks should lift off the floor. **1**

> Now slowly roll back to the start position; your legs are once again stretched upwards.

> **Advanced:** Those of you who are in good condition can try the following extension to the exercise:

> Start position: as before.

> Stretch your feet towards the ceiling so that your bottom lifts off the floor. **2**

> Now slowly roll back to the start position.

Important: It is especially important in this exercise that you work without force and do not use your body's momentum to push the movement. Otherwise you will overload your spine.

Leg roll

> Lying on your back, pull both thighs in toward your body. The angle between your upper body and thighs should be less than 90 degrees. Lay your arms out to the sides, bent at the elbows so that your finger-tips are pointing towards the ceiling and your elbows are almost at shoulder level.

> Press your upper arms into the floor with some force and hold this tension throughout the whole exercise. Now slowly lower your bent legs to the right, but only as far as you can with both shoulder blades still touching the floor. **3**

> Then lift the legs back to the center position. Repeat the motion going to the left and bring your legs back to the center again.

> **Advanced:** The exercise is made more difficult if the angle between your upper body and thighs is greater than 90 degrees.

Pendulum

> Lie with your back on the mat. Place your hands under your head. Pull your legs in toward your body, bent at the knee.

> Lift your head and roll your upper body off the floor. At the same time, stretch your right arm back over your head and move your left leg forward, bringing your left hand toward your right foot. **4**

> From here, reverse the movement slowly: Pull the left leg back toward your body and bring the right leg and arm forward.

3 | 8 times | 3 sets

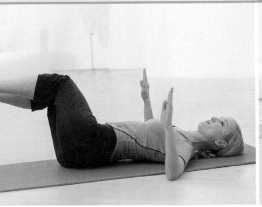

4 | 8 times | 3 sets

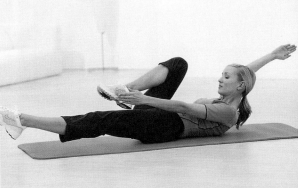

Twisted crunch

> Lie on your back on the mat. Place your left foot on the floor. Lay your right calf on your left thigh. Your left hand should be under your ear, the thumb resting on your temple or cheek bone so that the elbow points outward. Your right arm should be stretched out pointing off to the side.

> Now slowly raise your upper body, bringing your left shoulder toward your right knee. Your elbow must remain turned to the outside so that the movement comes only from your shoulder. Hold this position for a short time. **1**

> Now slowly lower yourself down to the mat.

> **Advanced:** The exercise is made more difficult if you keep both hands behind your head.

> A further step for advanced fitness practitioners: Place a weight on the upper shoulder and hold this in place with your free hand. **2**

1 **10 times per side | 3 sets**

2

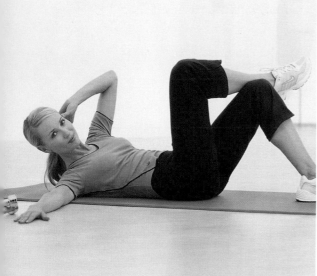

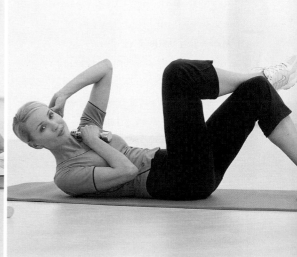

94

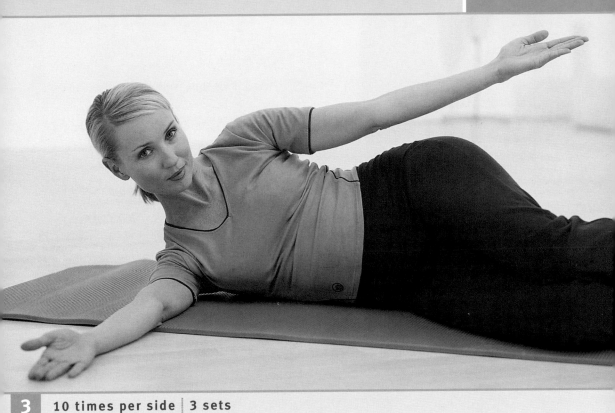

3 | **10 times per side** | **3 sets**

Side lift

> Lie on the mat on your right side. Gently bend your legs. Now stretch out your right arm along the floor, palm up. Stretch your left arm out parallel to your body pointed slightly upwards. The left hand should also be palm up.

> With your left hand, slowly push towards your feet so that your upper body lifts off the floor. **3**

> Now slowly lower your upper body back down to the mat.

> **Variation:** If it is more comfortable for you, you can also rest your left hand on your right shoulder during this exercise.

GET "CRUNCHY" IN THE OFFICE

TIP

Your stomach muscles often lead a shadowy existence during the day. Make them work: while sitting down, draw your navel inwards and press your back firmly into the chair back rest. Imagine that your ribs are pulling in toward your navel. Hold for around 10 seconds and release. Repeat 3–5 times.

Lower back

Diagonal lift from face-down position

> Lie on your stomach on the mat. Place your toes on the floor. Bend your right arm and lay your forehead on your right hand. Stretch your left arm out forward. Keep looking towards the floor throughout the exercise so that your neck remains relaxed.

> Now firmly tense your buttocks; this should lift your knees a little off the floor. Slowly raise the left arm just over the floor, turning your left thumb towards the ceiling. **1**

> Now raise your right leg slightly off the floor until you feel a stretch running diagonally across your body. **2**

> Hold this position for about 15 seconds, then lower your arm and leg to the floor.

1   4 times each side

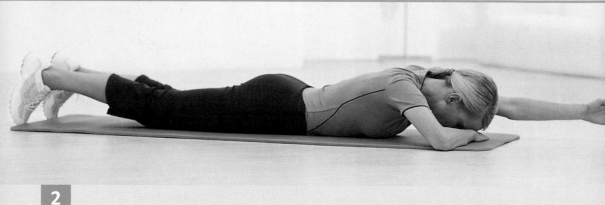

2

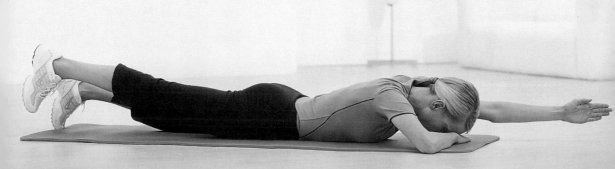

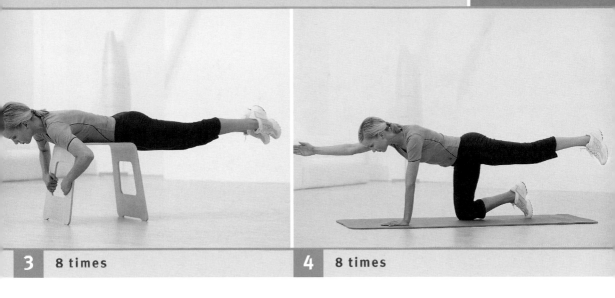

3	8 times	**4**	8 times

Double-sided leg lift

> Lie with your stomach on a stool so that your legs can move freely. Hold on tightly to the legs of the stool. Keep looking toward the floor.

> Now slowly raise both legs and stretch them out straight. Do not raise them higher than your back! **3**

> Hold your legs here for about 15 seconds and then slowly lower them to the floor.

Diagonal lift

> Kneel on all fours on the mat. The knees should be directly below the hip joints and the hands below the shoulders. But don't lock your elbows.

> Now slowly stretch your right arm out forward with the thumb facing toward the ceiling. Stretch your left leg out backwards. **4**

> Hold the position for around 10 seconds and then lower the arm and leg. Now do exactly the same with the opposing limbs.

> **Variation:** If you experience too much pressure on your knees in this position, roll your mat into a cushion.

Stretching and relaxing

Stretching out

> Lie on your back on the mat and stretch your arms above your head. Let your legs relax completely.
> Push your arms "out of your body" over your head until you feel a stretch in your stomach muscles. Now inhale very deeply and regularly (allow your abdomen to relax completely and expand) and exhale (your abdomen sinks). **1**
> In between, relax your arms each time and then stretch again. Do the exercise enough times until you feel it is doing you good.

Upper abdominal region

> Lay a rolled up towel on the floor. Lie on your back on the towel with your arms stretched above your head, so that your chest is pushed slightly upwards.
> Stretch your arms out above your head until you feel a stretch in the upper abdominal region. **2**
> Hold the stretch for around 15 seconds, then relax again.

1 several times

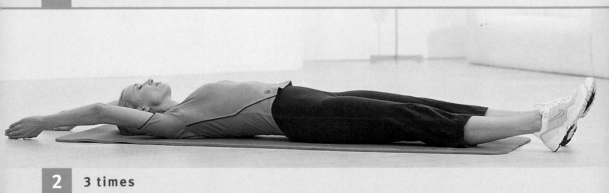

2 3 times

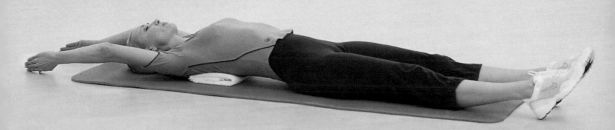

Lower back

> Kneel on the mat on all fours. Arms and thighs should be roughly perpendicular to the floor.
> Go into a "cat stretch": Pull your navel in toward your back so that your back is quite rounded. Allow your head to simply hang loosely. **3**
> Hold this position for around 15 seconds and then return to the start position.

Whole back

> Sit on the mat. Place your feet on the mat and place your hands in the crooks of your knees. Keep your back straight.
> Now move your upper body backwards in a slow, "rounding" movement. You should feel your spine rolling down, vertebra by vertebra. Go back as far as you need to so that all of your upper body weight is supported by your arms. Allow your head to simply hang loosely forward. **4**
> Hold this position for around 15 seconds and return to the start position.

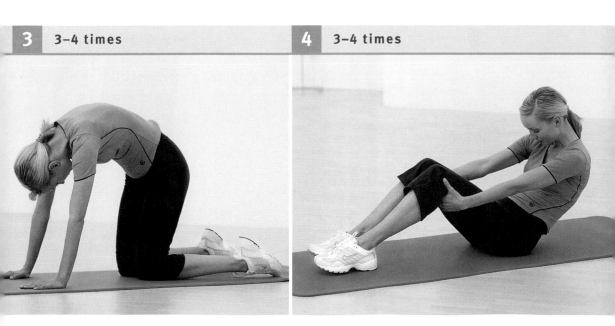

3 3–4 times

4 3–4 times

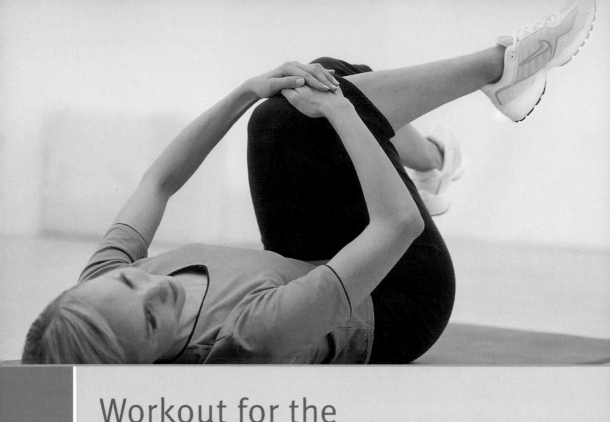

Workout for the lower body

A taut behind and slim, shapely legs are something wonderful. Unfortunately, with increasing age they represent real problem areas. The connective tissue becomes weaker and, at the same time, more fat is stored in these areas. As described on page 14, though, you do not have to resign yourself to these changes! With the correct exercise for your lower body you can continue to be pleased with your toned, slim shape for a long time yet.

The lower body workout is not only good for your looks but also for your health: Well-toned thigh muscles relieve and stabilize the knees, which take a lot of strain.

Well-toned buttocks make a significant contribution to good posture and the same is true for the muscles of the pelvic floor; firm, taut calves finally give you a good stance and are, especially in summer, a real head-turner!

Muscle groups of the lower body

Versatile: The thighs

Using the exercises from page 104 onward you can tone up all the muscles of the thighs: front and back (quadriceps and hamstrings) as well as inside and outside (adductors and abductors). After 40 it is particularly important to tone the muscles of the outer thigh since increased fat deposits tend to gather here. However, there is frequent misunderstanding of which muscles actually make up the outer thigh and how they can be exercised. So exercises which would in fact have a real effect on the appearance of the outer thighs may get overlooked.

(Often unequal) opposites

The outer thigh musculature is formed by the sartorius muscle and the outer parts of the quadriceps and hamstrings. While we use the quadriceps, the muscles at the front of the thigh, in almost all activities, its partner muscle at the back of the thigh, the hamstring, is usually not as active and is therefore less well-developed.

Quadriceps and hamstrings are therefore – alongside the abductors and adductors – very important for excercising the legs.

"Squats" (all kinds of knee-bending exercises) ensure, among other things, well-toned, firm outer thighs.

The backside needs exercise

The muscles of the buttocks usually get a raw deal. Normally they are rather neglected: through long periods of sitting in the office, in the car, in front of the television. The buttocks are surrounded by fatty tissue with very poor blood supply and the connective tissue in this area is extremely elastic. This means that without exercise it gets very slack. This makes the buttocks a prime candidate for cellulite (see page 14). At the same time it is very undemanding and is quite satisfied with regular, short exercises.

Well-exercised muscles in this area are not only nice to look at, they also support a healthy upright posture which relieves the joints. These muscles support the pelvis and are also responsible for stabilising the hips. The biggest and most important of the muscles of the buttocks is the gluteus maximus. It keeps the pelvis straight and is therefore responsible for the straightening of the hip joint. In addition, it ensures that the upper body does not lean forward when standing. Putting it all more succinctly, it is one of the main muscles responsible for good posture!

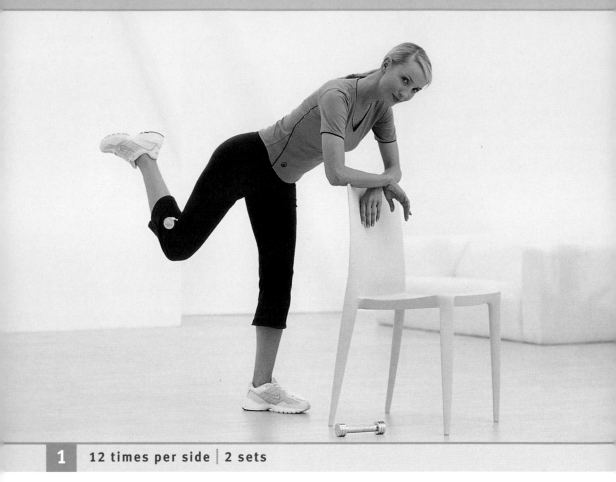

1 | **12 times per side | 2 sets**

Muscles of the buttocks

Kickbacks

> Stand behind a chair with a backrest. Bend your right leg behind you and lay a weight in the hollow of your right knee. Grip the weight between thigh and calf. Rest your forearms on the back of your chair. Keep your back straight and your gaze towards the floor. The left leg should be gently bent. Both knees should be side by side.
> Now slowly push the right leg with the weight backwards, consciously tensing your right buttock. Only lift the right leg as far as you can with a straight back. Don't allow the back to hollow! Hold this position for a short time. **1**
> Now slowly lower your leg to the start position.

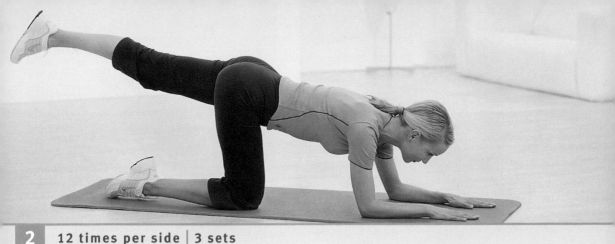

2   12 times per side | 3 sets

Leg lift

> Kneel on all fours on the mat and support yourself on your forearms, keeping your elbows under your shoulders and your knees under your hips. Hold your head loosely to stretch the spine out straight. Stretch the left leg out backwards until the toes are just touching the floor.

> Slowly lift the left leg until it is at the height of your back. **2**

> Then slowly lower the leg. Stop just above the floor and lift again.

Leg lift with stool

> Lie with your stomach on a stool so that your legs are free to move. Your neck should be straight and your gaze should be directed at the floor. Hold on to the stool with your hands.

> Slowly lift your right leg off the floor and stretch it out, raising it no further than your back. Hold briefly. **3**

> Now slowly lower the leg back to the floor.

3   12 times per side | 3 sets

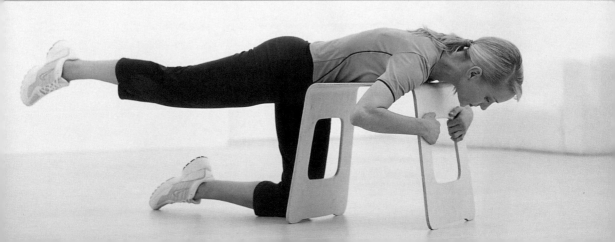

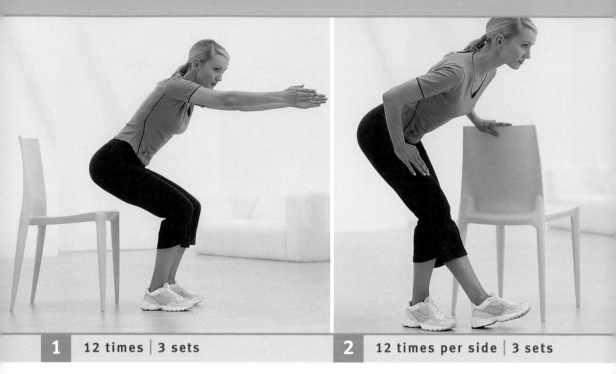

1   12 times | 3 sets   **2**   12 times per side | 3 sets

Buttocks and thighs

Knee bends (squats)

> Stand at a little more than a foot-
length from a chair. Your feet should
be parallel or make a slight "v"-shape
and at least hip-width apart. Transfer
your weight onto your heels so that
your toes lift slightly.

> Slowly push your buttocks backwards.
In order to keep your balance, stretch
your arms out in front. Stop just
before your buttocks touch the chair.
1

> Now slowly push your body weight
upwards again until your legs are
almost straight.

> **Advanced:** If you can do this exercise
easily, once you have lowered your
buttocks down you can gently bounce
three times before coming up again.
Or: Perform the exercise with weights.

One-legged squats

> Stand next to a chair with a backrest so
that you can hold onto it with your left
hand. Place your left heel about half a
foot-length in front of the right so that
your weight is now almost entirely
resting on your right leg.

> Support your right hand on your right
thigh and transfer your weight onto
your right heel. From this position push
your buttocks backwards. **2**

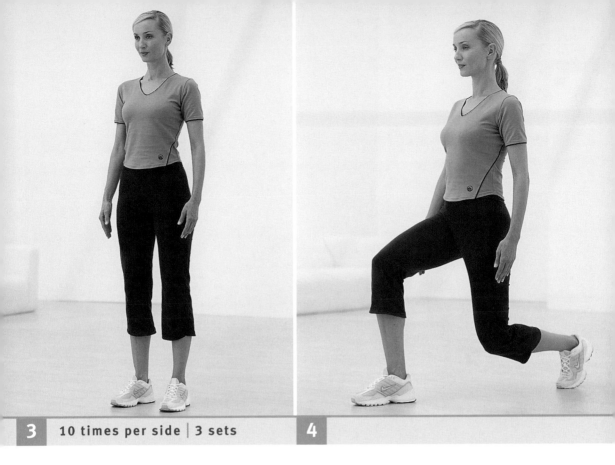

3   10 times per side | 3 sets   **4**

> Now slowly come back up.
> **Advanced:** If you can do this exercise easily, once you have lowered your buttocks down you can gently bounce three times before coming back up.

Lunge

> Stand with your legs about hip-width apart. Let your arms hang loosely down with the fingertips pointing towards the floor. **3**
> Take a big step forward with your right leg and place your whole foot flat on the floor.

> Now bend both legs further so that your bottom moves straight downward. The right knee should stay above your right heel, the left knee should move in the direction of the floor. **4**
> Now move back up to the start position. As you raise your right knee your right heel should be the last thing to leave the floor.
> **Advanced:** To make the exercise more difficult you can hold a weight in each hand.

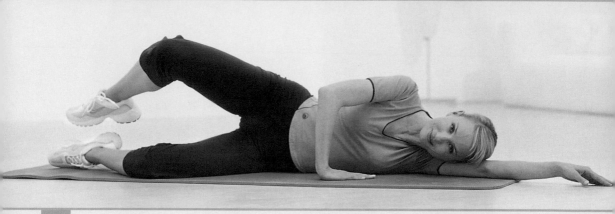

1 10 times per side | 2 sets

Abductor twists

> Lie on the mat on your left side. Stretch your left arm above your head and lay your head on your arm. Bend both legs. The angle between upper body and thighs should be greater than 90 degrees. Place your right hand on the floor in front of your chest. Lie so that shoulders and hips remain straight and do not tip to the side.

> Now gently raise your right leg. From this position lower your right heel to the left heel until your heels are touching; the knee should turn towards the ceiling as you do this. **1**

> Now turn the right leg so that the knees touch. **2**

> Then bring the heels together again.

2

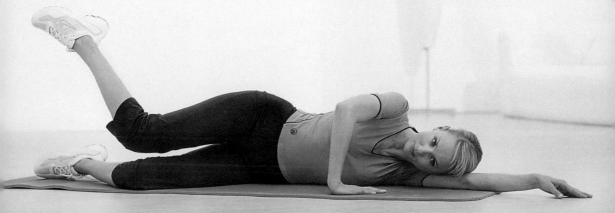

Abductors – on the side

> Lie on the mat on your right side. Bend your knees slightly so that the angle between upper body and thighs is greater than 90 degrees. Take a weight in your left hand and lay it on your left thigh. Now place your upper right arm on the floor. Rest your head in your right hand.

> Slowly lift your left leg. **3**

> Lower your leg to the start position.

Important: Make sure that you keep your body in a straight line and do not tip forwards or backwards.

Adductors – on the side

> Fold up a towel and lay it near your mat. Lie on your right side on the mat. Stretch your right arm above your head and rest your head on your arm. Now straighten out your right leg completely. Bend your left leg and rest your knee on the folded towel in front of you. Bend the leg as much as is comfortable for you. Place your left hand in front of your chest.

> Now raise the straight lower leg up off the floor. **4**

> Slowly lower your leg. Stop just above the floor and then raise it again.

Important: Make sure throughout this exercise that your pelvis remains straight and does not tip forwards or backwards.

3 10 times per side | 2 sets

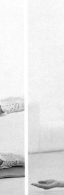

4 10 times per side | 2 sets

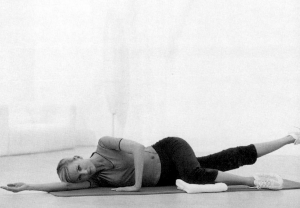

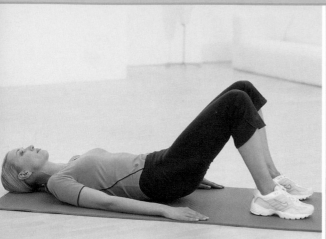

1 | 5 times

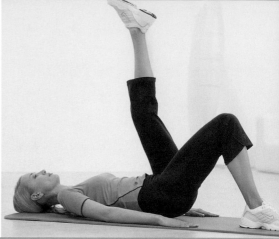

2 | 4 times per side

Pelvic floor

Pelvic tilt

> Lie with your back on the mat. Place your feet about hip-width apart on the floor. Your arms should be relaxed by your sides. To start, just consciously breathe in and out a couple of times.

> Now on the exhale, tense your pelvic floor muscles as if you wanted to stop urinating mid-stream. At the same time pull in your vaginal muscle so that your pubic bone moves slightly up towards your navel. The more intensively you exhale, the stronger you should tense these muscles. **1**

> Hold this tension for around 5 seconds, then relax. Before repeating, breathe deeply in and out 2 or 3 times.

Pelvic tilt with leg stretch

> Just like the previous exercise, lie on your back and place your feet about hip-width apart, your arms relaxed at your sides.

> Just like the "pelvic tilt", build up the tension on the exhale. Then stretch one leg up from the knee. The movement should come from just this one leg. Don't allow the other leg to help! **2**

> On the inhale slowly lower the leg again and relax the tension. Before changing legs breathe deeply in and out 2 or 3 times.

Calves

Double heel lifts

> Stand with your legs about hip-width apart behind a chair and hold on to the chair's backrest.
> Slowly raise your heels so that you are standing on the balls of your feet. Tense your calves at the same time. **3**
> Hold this tension for about 3 seconds, then slowly lower your heels back to the floor.

Single heel lifts

> Stand next to a chair so that you can hold onto the backrest with your right hand. Place your left foot on your right calf.
> Lift up onto the ball of your right foot and tense your calf. **4**
> Hold the tension for about 3 seconds, then slowly lower your heel to the floor.
> **Advanced:** To make the exercise more difficult hold a weight in your free hand.

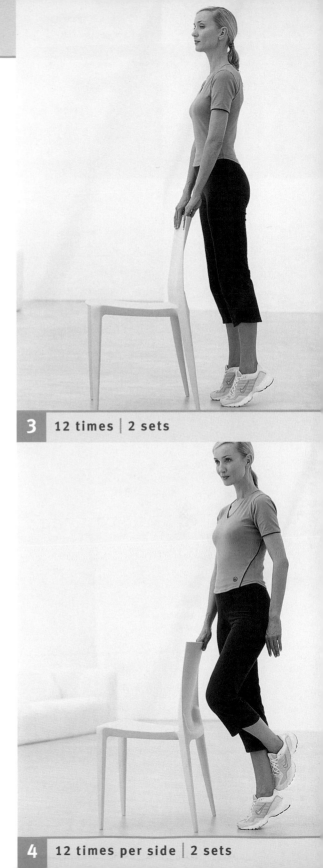

3 12 times | 2 sets

4 12 times per side | 2 sets

Stretching and relaxing

Abductors

> Stand next to a chair so that you can support yourself with your left hand on the backrest.
> Now cross your right calf over the front of your left thigh. Place your right hand on your right thigh and bring your upper body forward and down. Push your buttocks backwards; your back should stay straight. **1**
> Hold this stretch for 10–15 seconds, then relax.

Quadriceps

> Stand near a chair so that you can support yourself with your left hand on the backrest.
> Slowly draw your right calf towards your buttocks and grasp your right ankle with your right hand. Move your thigh slowly backwards until it is parallel to your left thigh. Now pull in your navel. **2**
> Hold this stretch for 10–15 seconds, then relax.

1 3 times per side

2 3 times per side

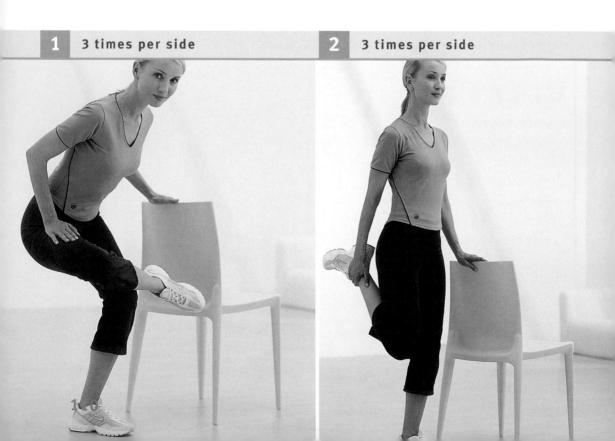

Backs of the thighs

> Lie with your back on the mat. Place your left heel on the floor and raise your right leg towards your body. Clasp your right thigh with both hands.
> Now slowly stretch your right leg as far as it will go and at the same time pull it toward your upper body. If possible, stretch your left leg out along the floor. **3**
> Hold this stretch for 10–15 seconds, then relax.
> **Variation:** This will be easier if you place a towel around the thigh and use it to pull your thigh towards your body. **4**

Important: Keep your shoulders completely relaxed.

Buttocks

> Lying on your back, draw your bent left leg towards your body.
> Now bring your right leg towards you as well, crossing your right thigh behind your left. Grasp both knees with your arms and pull them towards your upper body until you feel a stretch in your buttocks. **5**
> Hold this stretch for 10–15 seconds, then relax. After three repetitions cross your legs the other way around.

Important: Keep your shoulders relaxed.

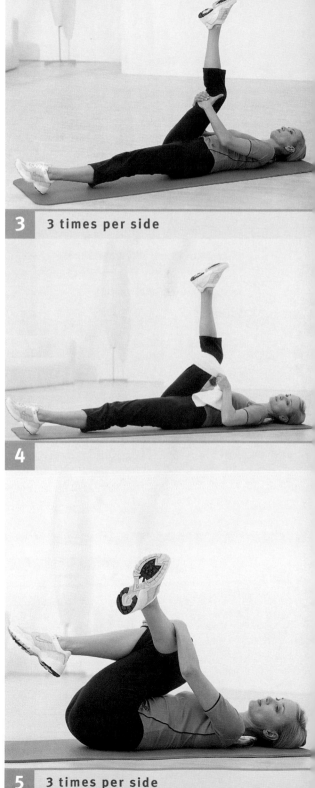

3 3 times per side

4

5 3 times per side

EXERCISING IN THE FITNESS STUDIO

With the help of this table you can put together an exercise program to use in the fitness studio that exactly fits your training plan. Here you will find exercises for use on equipment in the studio that correspond to the exercises in the book; the same muscle groups will be exercised using similar movements.

For some of the exercises in the book there are no particular pieces of equipment to be found in the studio – for example for the core stability exercises. In this case, suitable exercises are those such as cable-pulley training in which all the muscles of the torso are involved.

Muscle groups of the upper body	
Exercise in book	Equipment/exercise in studio
Upper back, especially rotators	
Rotators with weight, p. 68	Rotator trainer with cable pull
Flying on your stomach, p. 70	Fly reverse with short weights
Whole upper back	
Rowing with weights, p. 68	Rowing machine
Apron strings, p. 70	Butterfly reverse
Chest muscles	
Pull-over, p. 72	Pull-over machine
Flying on your back, p. 73	Butterfly
Push-ups, pp. 74, 75	Seated chest press
Shoulder muscles	
Side arm raises, p. 76	Side lift machine
Forward arm raises, p. 76	Front lift with cable pull
Overhead press, S. 77	Shoulder press
Arm muscles – triceps	
Arm stretches, p. 78	Triceps machine
Dips, pp. 78, 79, 80	Dip trainer with/without support
Arm muscles – biceps	
Biceps: Hammer curls, p. 80	Biceps machine
Biceps curl, one-sided, p. 81	Biceps curl with short/long weight

Muscle groups of the mid-section

Exercise in book	Equipment/exercise in studio
Whole mid-section	
Balance, p. 88	Stabilisation exercises at the cable pull
Shoulder push-up, p. 88	Stabilisation exercises at the cable pull
Long support, p. 89	Stabilisation exercises at the cable pull
Rectus abdominus muscles	
Basic crunch, p. 90	Seated abdominal trainer
Knee crunch, p. 91	Reverse abdominal trainer
Leg dips, p. 91	Reverse abdominal trainer
Pelvic roll, p. 92	Reverse abdominal trainer
Obliques	
Leg roll, p. 93	Torso rotation machine
Pendulum, p. 93	Torso rotation machine with cable pull
Twisted crunch, p. 94	Torso rotation machine
Side lift, p. 95	Side bends on the bench
Lower back	
Diagonal lift, face down, p. 96	Back bench
Double-sided leg lift, p. 97	Hip-stretch machine
Diagonal lift, p. 97	Back stretch machine

Muscle groups of the lower body

Exercise in book	Equipment/exercise in studio
Bottom muscles	
Kick backs, p. 102	Hip stretch with cable pull
Leg lift, p. 103	Leg stretch with cable pull
Leg lift with stool, p. 103	Hip stretch machine
Buttock and thigh muscles	
Knee bends (squats), p. 104	Leg press, seated or lying
One-legged squats, p. 104	Squats with long or short weight
Lunge, p. 105	Lunges with short weight
Abductors	
Abductor twists. p.106	Abductor trainer with cable pull
Abductors – on the side, p. 107	Abductor machine, seated
Inside of the thigh	
Adductors – on the side, p. 107	Abductor machine, seated
Calf muscles	
Double heel lifts, p. 109	Calf trainer, seated
Single heel lifts, p. 109	Calf raises with short weights

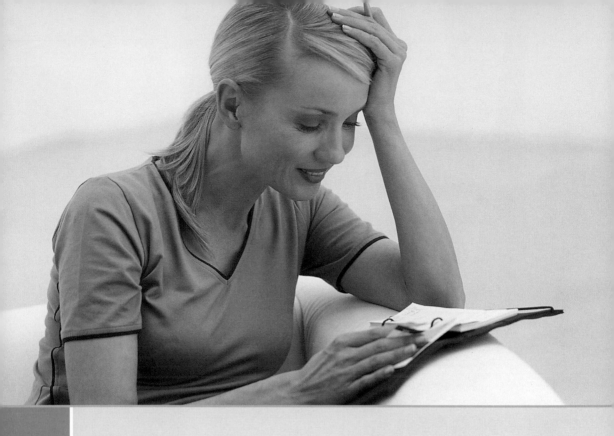

Turbo workout and weekly training plan

Just one form of exercise that stays fun and can be planned into your day without causing you stress can guarantee that you really stick with it. Simply put: if you have never done regular exercise up until now it can be difficult to get started, and not necessarily because you can't be bothered. Perhaps you just don't know how to put together an exercise program that will suit your personal training needs as well as your daily routine. All of the different exercises and possibilities for stamina training can be a little overwhelming. In order to make it easier to get started and to give you examples of how you can plan your exercise, over the next few pages there is the 10-minute workout program for those people who are in a hurry and two exercise programs for your all-over workout for the whole week.

10-minute turbo workout

Exercising for 10 minutes every day – does it get you anywhere? You'll be amazed! After only one hour of exercise a week in total, our bodies begin to build up muscle. It works all the better if several muscle groups are challenged at once in each exercise, in small "chunks" of exercise – as shown in the 10-minute turbo workout on the next pages.

Even if regular exercise is already a part of your daily routine, situations can arise in which you would like to go for a small, quick exercise session – for example when traveling or if you have visitors. For those times when you have a sudden period of high stress it is also a good idea to have a well-planned "emergency program" in place. And what a shame it would be if the progress you had made so far were to go to waste because of taking too long a break from exercise!

With the program on the following pages you can get going at any time. And the nice thing about it – it's just like a good meal, a little taste whets your appetite for more. It's true! Here's something that many people experience: if your body gets a taste for exercise through regular training it will certainly demand more. So your workout becomes just as much a pleasure and reward as food and drink.

YOU SHOULD ALWAYS MAKE TIME FOR THIS

When you are feeling particularly stressed and you have a workout planned in your schedule, you should perform the exercises slowly and consciously, as usual, and make sure that you breathe deeply and evenly while doing them.
Warming up and cooling down are always part of a successful exercise session, that will leave you feeling fit and relaxed. In the end this will benefit you in your other daily activities as well!

IMPORTANT !

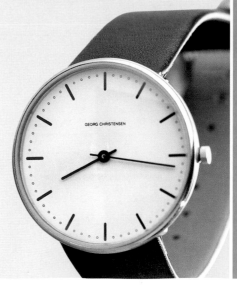

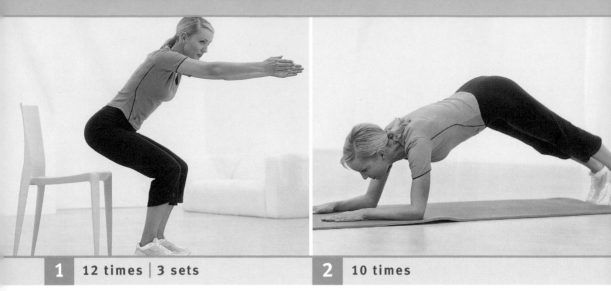

1 | 12 times | 3 sets

2 | 10 times

Knee bends (squats)

With this exercise you will train the muscles of the front and back of the thighs as well as the buttocks (page 104).
1

Long support

The long support with dip trains the whole musculature of the torso – the muscles of the upper and lower back as well as the abdominal muscles (page 89). **2**

Twisted crunch

With this exercise it is mainly the oblique abdominals and also the rectus abdominus muscles that are strengthened (page 94). **3**

Push-ups

With push-ups you are training the arm and chest muscles and the upper back. Choose the appropriate difficulty level (page 74). **4**

3 | 10 times per side | 3 sets

4 | 10 times | 2 sets

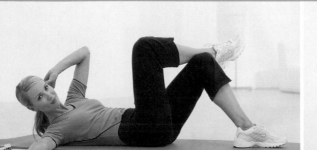

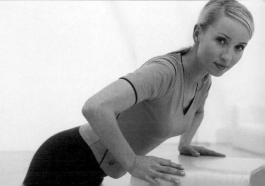

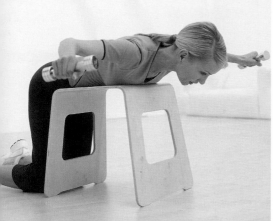

5 12 times | 2 sets

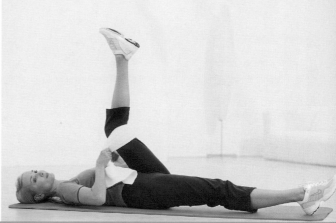

6 3 times per side

Flying on your stomach

An exercise for the upper back, especially the rotators, should be in every workout program (page 70). **5**

Hamstrings (Stretch)

Choose the exercise method with which you feel most comfortable (page 111). **6**

Chest stretch

Try both variations (page 85). **7**

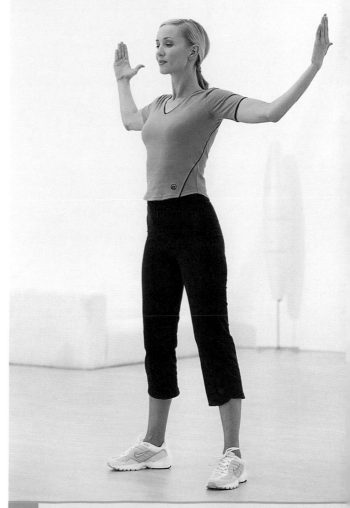

7 3 times

Weekly training plan

In order to effectively exercise the whole body and all muscle groups you need a well-balanced exercise program. On this and the following pages you will find two example programs, which should each be performed twice a week. This means you can exercise your whole body with four sessions a week.

Of course, you can also put together your own exercise program. With a little workout experience this will come to you very easily.

Program I: Upper body and abdomen

Rotators with weight
For the upper back (page 68) **1**

Push-ups
For chest muscles, arms and upper back. Choose your own difficulty level (pages 74/75) **2**

Flying on your stomach
For the upper back (page 70) **3**

Side arm raises
For the shoulder muscles (page 76) **4**

One-sided biceps curl
For the front of the arms (page81) **5**

Dips
For the upper-arm muscles (page 78) **6**

Long support
For the whole torso (page 89) **7**

Twisted crunch
For the obliques and the rectus abdominus muscles (page 94) **8**

Stretches to finish

Upper abdominal area
For the rectus abdominus muscles (page 98) **9**

Chest
Choose one of the stretches for the chest area (page 85) **10**

Neck
To loosen the neck area (page 84) **11**

TIP

EXAMPLE OF AN OPTIMAL EXERCISE PLAN

Program I: Program II:	Upper body and abdomen Lower body and abdomen
Monday	Program I
Tuesday	Program II
Wednesday	Rest or stamina training (see page 42)
Thursday	Program I
Friday	Program II
Saturday or **Sunday**	Stamina training again

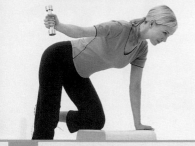

1   12 times/side | 2 sets

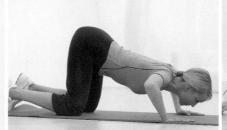

2   10 times | 2 sets

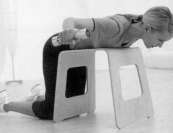

3   12 times | 2 sets

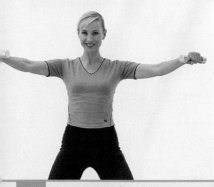
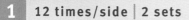

4   10 times | 2 sets

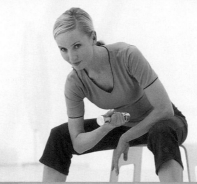

5   12 times/Seite | 2 sets

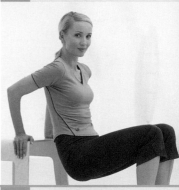

6   12 times | 2 sets

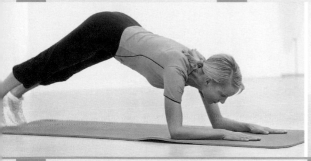

7   10 times

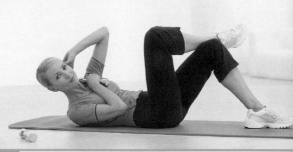

8   10 times per side | 3 sets

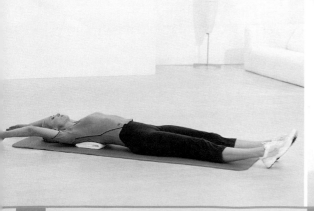

9   3 times

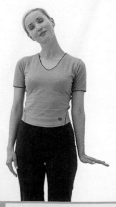

10   3 times

11   3 times

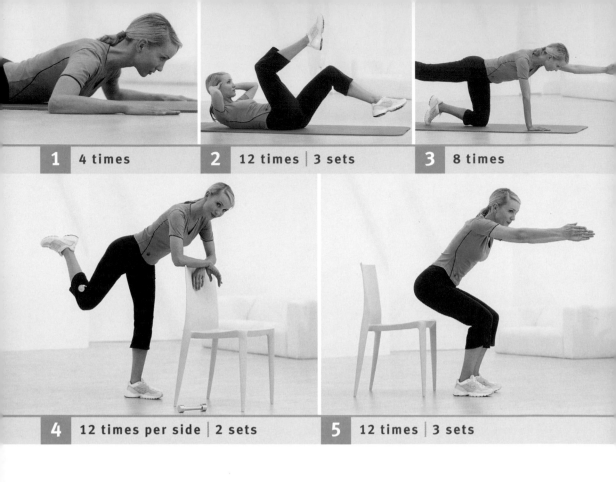

1 4 times	**2** 12 times | 3 sets	**3** 8 times
4 12 times per side | 2 sets	**5** 12 times | 3 sets	

Program II: Lower body and abdomen

Shoulder push-up
For the whole torso musculature (page 88)

Leg lowering
For the abdominals (page 91) 2

Diagonal lift
For the back extender muscles (page 97)
3

Kickbacks
For the buttock muscles (page 102) 4

Knee bends (squats)
For the fronts and backs of the thighs
including the outer thighs (page 104) 5

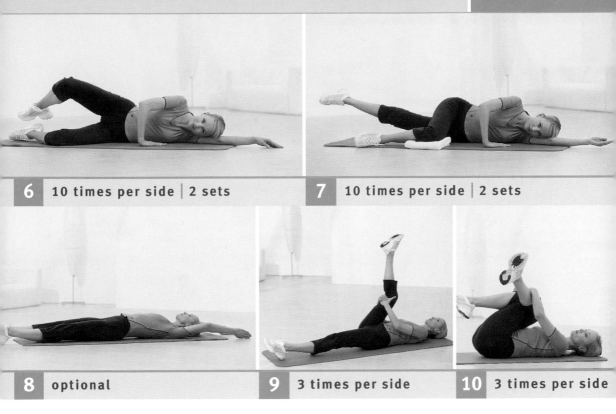

6 10 times per side | 2 sets

7 10 times per side | 2 sets

8 optional

9 3 times per side

10 3 times per side

Abductor twist
For the muscles of the outer thighs
(page 106) **6**

Adductor – on the side
For the muscles of the inner thighs
(page 107) **7**

Stretches

Stretching out
For the rectus abdominus (page 98) **8**

Hamstrings
For the muscles on the backs of the
thighs (page 111) **9**

Bottom
For the buttock muscles (page 111) **10**

Index

Index of exercises

The most important points at a glance

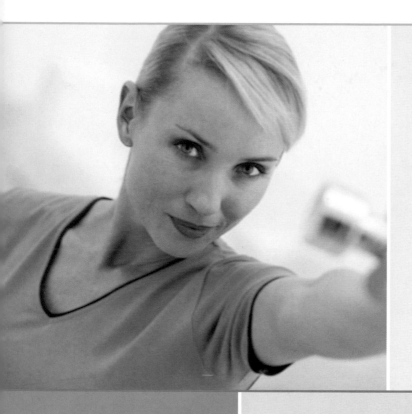

The quartet of success

Strength and stamina, mobility and coordination are the four pillars of your fitness. They can only be strong together! Combine the exercises in this book with what the fitness studios or sports clubs have to offer; that way you will be able to put together your ideal exercise program.

MUSCLES WORK BEST IN HARMONY

A posture that is straight and kind to joints and back, an attractive figure – these will not come about by gaining impressive muscle bulk but with building a balanced relationship of strengths. That's the only way to get all of your muscle groups to work together harmoniously. Pay particular attention to your mid-section as you do this since the muscles here are important for supporting the body and respond very well to training, particularly in women.

WARM UP – GET GOING – RELAX

Targeted warm-up and stretching exercises are a part of every well-planned training session. Warming up switches your body into "activity mode". Stretching protects your body from strains and injuries, prevents aching muscles and increases the positive effects of your training. The gentle pulling makes the muscles nice and supple and just feels good! There are two different techniques which can be used – static and dynamic stretching, which you can use according to your own needs.

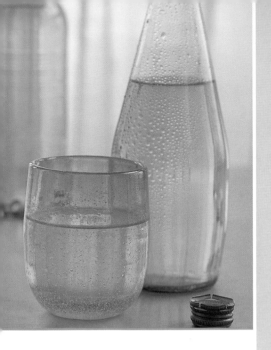

BAD TIMES FOR EXCESS FAT

The most effective way to get your metabolism going is with measured stamina training. Then the body can tap into its fat reserves and will store less. Because you are also building up your muscles with a regular workout, your body will burn more fat, even at rest. Of course, diet also plays a role: Carbohydrates from whole-grain, high-value proteins and sensible amounts of healthy fats and oils, as well as plenty of vitamins and minerals are the ideal basis for your Bodystyling menu.

It's all in the planning

With very little effort you can put together your own fitness plan which is perfectly suited to your needs. That way you'll have a successful program which fits your day-to-day life. The tips and exercise programs in this Advice Guide will help you accomplish this.

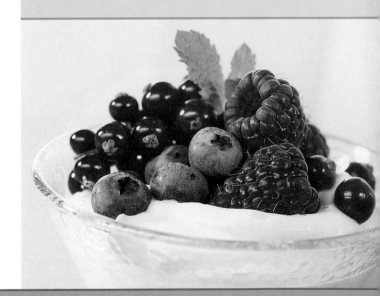

DON'T FORGET TO TOP OFF YOUR TANKS!

Water is as important to the body as oxygen. Your body can only properly function when it has enough water at its disposal. One half-gallon of water, fruit juice and water combined or herbal tea should be the least you take on board during the day. Apart from this, drinking also helps you lose weight as it quells hunger pangs and cleanses waste products from your system.

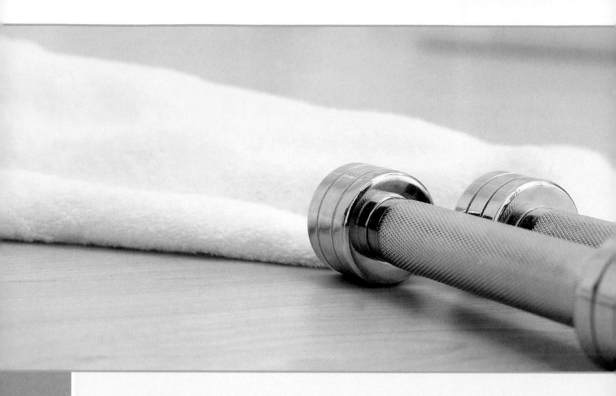

Jutta Schuhn is a graduate sports teacher and dance therapist with more than fifteen years' experience as an instructor, education leader and top international demonstrator/advisor for numerous leading sporting goods manufacturers. Among other commendations, she was awarded "Demonstrator of the Year 1998" and "Euro-Star 1999". Jutta Schuhn has also written and co-written numerous books and magazine articles on the subject. Being over 40 herself, she understands the particular demands of this time of life.

Elmar Trunz-Carlisi is a sports scientist who heads the Institute for Prevention and Care in Cologne. He specialises in fitness and sport for health and has numerous publications in this field to his name in all forms of media: general interest and specialist magazines, books and television contributions, scientific publications. Elmar Trunz-Carlisi has been an advisor and producer for the specialist fitness magazine "Bodylife" for over 10 years and since 1996 has been a member of the European team for the fitness magazine "Fit for Fun".